THE

PRISON

DOCTOR

Dr Amanda Brown is a GP at the largest women-only prison in Europe, Bronzefield. She was a regular NHS GP for a number of years, until she gave up her practice to move into the prison service. She worked at a teenage detention centre, before moving on to Wormwood Scrubs and then finally to Bronzefield where she continues to practice to this day. *The Prison Doctor* is her first book.

THE

PRISON

DOCTOR

My time inside Britain's
most notorious jails.

DR AMANDA BROWN

with Ruth Kelly

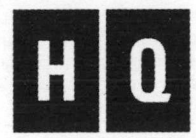

ONE PLACE. MANY STORIES

In loving memory of my beloved mother and father who taught me the true meaning of the words love and compassion a very long time ago.

HQ
An imprint of HarperCollinsPublishers Ltd.
1 London Bridge Street
London SE1 9GF

This edition 2019

9
First published in Great Britain by
HQ, an imprint of HarperCollinsPublishers Ltd. 2019

ISBN: 978-0-00-831144-5

MIX
Paper from
responsible sources
FSC
www.fsc.org
FSC™ C007454

This book is produced from independently certified FSC paper to ensure responsible forest management.

For more information visit: www.harpercollins.co.uk/green

This book is set in 11.2/16 pt. Sabon

Printed and bound by
CPI Group, Croydon CR0 4YY

Since writing this book the prescribing policy in Bronzefield has changed, and it is no longer permitted for any doctor to prescribe pregabalin to support withdrawal from illicit use. The tally system for collecting prison keys has been replaced by a TRAKA system

Contents

'The mind is its own place and in itself can make a Heaven of Hell, a Hell of Heaven.'

– JOHN MILTON, *Paradise Lost*

Prologue

HMP Bronzefield

I arrived to shouting and screaming. Prison officers were sprinting across the corridor and up the metal stairs.

'What's happening?' I shouted, thinking a fight must have broken out.

I've seen and heard a lot during my fifteen years as a prison doctor, but the reply shocked me.

'Someone's having a baby!' one of the officers yelled, repeating the news into his radio. He called for back-up, an ambulance, nurses, for all medical staff to come to House Block One.

'*Oh bloody hell!*'

I followed the stampede. We sounded like a small army trampling up the metal stairs.

The deep stench of overcooked vegetables from lunch lingered in the air, green and ripe, sweet and rotten, mixed with sweat and cheap soap.

The prisoners heard us coming, thumping their fists on their cell doors. Metal thunder, filling the air.

Half a dozen officers were already crowded outside the entrance to the tiny cell at the end.

'Coming through!' I said, squeezing past them.

A shaft of light poured through the small barred window. Hiding in the shadows of the corner was a tiny young woman, standing and shaking. Her nightie was soaked in blood from the waist down. The walls were splattered too; violent red sprays, like protest graffiti.

She looked completely shell-shocked. In that moment, she didn't know where or who she was. Her wiry black hair was drenched in sweat and glued across her face.

But where was the baby?

I tried to appear calm, stepping closer, trying to reassure her.

'Hi, sweetheart, you're going to be okay.'

Who knew if that were true? I suspected the prisoner was a heroin addict currently on methadone. The majority of prisoners on House Block One had a history of substance misuse.

The banging of the doors grew louder. Shouting and swearing, the air full of heat and sound and pressure. When the prison was like that it felt as if a spark could blow the place sky high.

The woman started screaming.

'Get it out of me! Get it out of me!'

She must have meant her placenta because there, partially hidden by the bed, lying in a pool of blood on the cold prison floor, was a tiny baby girl.

I looked around, trying to see something I could use to wrap her up. The umbilical cord was torn, presumably ripped apart by her mother. The baby was so small I suspected she was a good few weeks premature. *But was she alive? Was this poor, poor girl ali—*

To my overwhelming relief she started to cry.

'Has anyone got any clean towels?' I asked.

'Here you go, Doc.' Becky, the prison officer, handed me the only clean thing she had to hand – a blue bed sheet.

I scooped her up into my arms, wrapped the prison sheets around her and held her close, desperately trying to warm up her fragile body. What a way to come into the world. She nestled into my chest and her crying settled a little.

I looked along the landing, desperately hoping for a sign of the ambulance. Both mother and baby needed to be transferred to hospital as soon as possible. The mother had clearly lost a lot of blood and as the placenta had not yet been delivered she was at risk of a postpartum haemorrhage, a major cause of maternal mortality.

While we waited, I checked for active bleeding. Thankfully there was no sign. But however relieved I felt, it was no comfort to her.

'Get it out of me! Get it out of me!' she continued to scream, over and over again, showing no interest at all in her baby. I worried she had not wanted the child, and wondered if she had been raped. I met so many women who had been the victims of gruesome sexual assaults.

The fear for the baby was that she may well have been subjected to drugs during the pregnancy. Any addictive substance that the mother may have used could also cause the foetus to become addicted. At birth the baby's dependence continues, but as the drug is no longer available symptoms of withdrawal can occur. This is known as neonatal abstinence syndrome. Symptoms can begin within twenty-four to forty-eight hours and require very careful management.

'Make room for the paramedics!' someone shouted, and relief washed over me as I heard the thumping of boots.

They came into the cell and one of the officers handed me a white towel for the baby. It might seem trivial in such a horrific situation, but I found a great deal of comfort in knowing that beautiful creation – with a mop of dark hair plastered to her head, a mirror of her mother – would be wrapped in a soft, warm towel rather than prison sheets.

The paramedics placed a blanket around the mother's shoulders and gently guided her into a wheelchair. She was still screaming 'Get it out of me!' as they started wheeling her away. She stared briefly at her baby in disbelief and disappeared from view.

Two prison officers would be needed to escort her to hospital, with one officer cuffed to the prisoner, just in case she tried to make a run for it. I didn't think I'd ever get over the sight of that, however much I knew it was necessary. I'd been taught that no prisoner is ever too sick to make a dash for freedom. The story of a new mum who jumped from the first floor window of a hospital maternity ward still does the rounds.

One of the paramedics turned to me, opening her arms: it was time to hand over the baby.

I gave the little girl one last cuddle, gently stroking her cheek with my forefinger. She wrapped her whole hand around my little finger and I said a little prayer in my head, hoping for the best.

If she was allowed to stay with her mum they would be located on the Mother and Baby Unit, on return from hospital, for a maximum of eighteen months. If the mother's sentence was longer, the child would then be taken into care. However, if it was decided the mother wasn't fit to care for her baby they would be separated very soon after birth.

Being a mother myself, I can't imagine what it must feel like to have your baby taken from you. To spend the days and nights in prison, imagining how she is growing up, what she looks like, who is taking care of her when she cries.

What would happen to the baby? I could look into it, of course. I could ask. I could follow the case through. But could I bear to know?

My contribution to the prisoners' lives is limited. I can't rewrite history for them, but I can take the edge off their suffering. I can help wean them off their addictions. I can be a listening ear.

My job is not to judge them but to care for them, and helping people, regardless of who they are and what they have done, is what I live for.

Everyone filed out and I was left alone, staring at the stained walls, the bloodied footprints. The claustrophobic grimness of the cell.

'You all right, Doc?' Becky asked.

'Yes, mate,' I sighed.

I followed her back downstairs and threw on my armour. It wasn't just the prisoners who needed to be strong to survive being in there. If I took everything I saw to heart, I'd be a mess.

I had a job to do – other people were waiting for me.

PART ONE

Where It All Began

2004–2009

Chapter One

'Wait up, Doc!' I spotted Gary, a prison officer, running towards me.

Many of the gates in the prison are alarmed, and staff have about thirty seconds to lock them before the sirens start blaring. I held the gate open. He weaved himself through in the nick of time.

I pulled the heavy gate shut, the resounding clang ringing through our ears. I locked it with one of the five keys chained to my black leather prison-issue belt. I knew which key I needed without looking; I've locked and unlocked those gates so many times.

We were in the central atrium at HMP Bronzefield. The largest female prison in Europe. Home to seventeen out of the twenty most dangerous women in the UK. Some high-profile murderers have been locked up here. Serial killer Joanna Dennehy, Becky Watts's killer Shauna Hoare, Mairead Philpott who helped start a fire that killed six of her children. Then there was Rosemary West, of course, also once a prisoner there – or 'resident' as they are referred to in Bronzefield.

The atrium roof is surrounded by windows; daylight, bright and beautiful, 60 feet above your head. In the middle of the room, five very tall synthetic trees reach towards the light. Even the plastic trees are trying to get out of there. It's bright and airy, a far cry from the tiny cells where the prisoners spend so much of their time.

'You're looking tanned!' I told him.

Gary grinned at the memory of his week of freedom.

'Seven days and six nights in Spain. All inclusive, the missus loved it. I didn't want to come back!'

But I knew that wouldn't be quite true. The shifts can be long and exhausting, physically and emotionally, but for some reason we do still want to turn up for work. And it's not just because it pays the bills.

It gets into your bones. The drama, the camaraderie, the highs and lows. I can honestly say I would rather spend a Friday evening working in Reception – meeting prisoners arriving from court, a diverse range of people, from different backgrounds, different cultures – than be out socialising.

But then, I'm not very good at small talk any more.

After hearing the sorts of stories I have over the years, I find it hard to engage in social chit-chat. I find it hard to talk about things that are trivial. You'd think I'd relish the break, the relief from the seriousness, but I don't think of it like that. Every day I'm part of something important. I think of it as an honour, a privilege, that people, often from completely different worlds from mine, will choose to confide in me and relate to me.

I don't know if it was his break away from the place, but Gary was in a philosophical mood. As we walked towards the gates which lead on to the Healthcare unit, our keys jangling with every footstep, he turned to me and said, 'You know what, Doc, I've been thinking.'

'Uh oh!' I teased him.

He flashed me a smile and then suddenly looked serious.

'I've been thinking about life. This place, and why people end up here.'

I was intrigued. 'Go on.'

Gary had been at HMP Bronzefield for fourteen years and was one of the good guys. He liked the challenge of dealing with the emotional needs of prisoners; he wanted to see them reformed.

He frowned, thinking for a moment. 'I think most prisoners have had a *Sliding Doors* moment,' he said. 'You know, that point in life where your life could really go either of two ways.'

I stood back while he opened the next set of gates. Like me, his fingers found the right key without ever having to look.

We made our way into the medical suite, a selection of rooms off a narrow corridor. I waved hello to Soheila in the pharmacy.

'It could happen to anyone, couldn't it?' he continued. 'A moment, a random moment when your whole life hangs in the balance. Like . . .' He tried to think of an example.

'You're having a drink in a pub, a fight breaks out, you hit someone, that person falls back and smacks their head. They die. The next thing you know, you're banged up inside for manslaughter.

'Your life can change in the blink of an eye. You know what I mean, Doc?'

Of course I knew. After all, it was just such a moment that had led to me being there.

Buckinghamshire
2004

The warmth of the central heating blasted into my face as I walked through the entrance doors of my GP practice.

I was greeted with a smile from Kirsty on reception.

'Morning, Amanda!'

I had no idea how she managed to be so cheerful, so early in the day.

As usual I felt daunted at the thought of how many patients I was likely to be seeing that day, but I loved my job as a GP – however exhausting it was.

I tugged my gloves off with my teeth, and picked up a pile of letters and notes Kirsty had put aside for me. So much paperwork.

'How's today looking?' I asked.

'Fully booked. Biscuit?' Kirsty waved the packet under my nose.

I shook my head. 'Don't forget the lunchtime meeting.'

'All scheduled, she said, tapping at the calendar on her computer screen with her biscuit.

My stomach somersaulted thinking of the meeting, and the changes it might bring to my cosy practice.

 In less than a month, on 1 April 2004, the new GP contract would be introduced, in which the whole pay structure for general practice would change. The basic pay would be reduced, but bonus payments could be earned if certain questions were asked and checks were done during the consultation.

I think it was intended to make GPs perform better, but I knew I'd struggle with it – gathering such information when perhaps a patient was deeply depressed or had recently been diagnosed with cancer, might feel inappropriate.

After twenty years my patients knew me too well. They would be able to see through why I was asking the questions, and I knew I couldn't do it just for the sake of it.

I reflected on how things had changed in the two decades since I'd started the surgery from scratch. The practice was within easy reach of London, and I'd managed to build my list up to about four thousand patients.

I'd moved with the times, always adapting to the changes within the health system and my surgery, but this latest scheme was threatening my core beliefs and principles concerning patient care. I was deeply concerned that I wouldn't be able to change my consultation style and gather the information required to earn the bonus payments. I also had a terrible inkling that my practice partners would demand I do so.

At 1 p.m. I steeled myself for what was to come, grabbed my note book and pen, and headed along the corridor to the meeting room.

Pretty pictures of landscapes, seascapes and flowers lined my way. I'd worked hard over the years to remove the sterile feel a new-build can have, to create a welcoming environment where people could feel relaxed. Small touches like that mattered to me.

I was the first to arrive.

I sat down to wait for the practice manager and my two partners, who now co-owned a share of the surgery. They were both excellent doctors, young and ambitious, and as I had never been particularly good at managing money or the business side of running the practice, I was more than happy to let them take charge.

The door swung open. Rohit, one of my GP partners, walked in, rubbing his hands. The other two followed close behind. They took their seats.

The tension was palpable. I sat there, legs crossed, anxiety building. My heart was pounding and I felt sick.

Rohit looked directly at me. 'So, how are you feeling about the changes, Amanda?' he asked.

We both had strong personalities and didn't always see eye to eye.

I leant forward, crossing my arms on the table. My shirt

tightened across my back, absurdly making me feel even more trapped.

Rohit leant back, giving me a tight little smile.

'Well . . .' I started, and didn't stop until I'd expressed how unhappy I felt about the new scheme. I was open and honest with them about what I was – and, most importantly, wasn't – prepared to do.

They glanced sideways at each other.

We were all silent for a while.

Rohit cleared his throat. 'Well, if you don't pull your weight financially, we will resent you,' he said in an icy tone.

I felt like the wind had been punched out of my lungs.

Resent *me*? I was the one who had built up the practice!

I felt furious. Unappreciated. But most of all, hurt.

Resent me? To be made to feel so worthless, to be expected to live with their resentment, or toe the line to make more money . . .

I couldn't work like this. I *wouldn't* work like this.

It was my *Sliding Doors* moment. In the blink of an eye, my life took an unexpected turn.

'Well, I'm leaving then,' I said.

All three stared at me in disbelief as I slowly peeled myself out of my chair and walked out of the door.

I must have looked white as a ghost, as Kirsty on reception asked if I was all right.

'No, I'm leaving.' I choked back tears.

I heard her gasp, but whatever words followed were lost

as I walked through the front doors, out into the cold. The wintery air hit my lungs, making it even harder to breathe.

What was I going to do now? I was forty-nine and turning my back on my career, my income, on *everything*.

I spun around and stared at the surgery I had created from nothing all those years ago. With it's pretty rhododendron hedge that I'd planted to give it a more welcoming, community feel. The building my property developer husband, David, had built for me. I thought about the thousands of patients on my list, many of whom had become like friends. I'd watched their children grow up, I'd listened to them when they worried, seen some make huge life changes. I'd held the hands of heartbroken elderly patients as they cried with loneliness. I hadn't been just a doctor: at times I felt as if I'd been a counsellor, a social worker, a vicar, a friend, all rolled into one. I had loved my life as a village GP, and over the years I had grown to know and love so many of the people I cared for that I used to joke I could write a book on many of them. Apart from my family, my surgery had been the most important thing in my life.

And just like that, it was all over.

*

I couldn't sleep.

I'd been staring at the same spot on the ceiling for hours. David held my hand while I lay there, chewing over my decision. My husband, my boys – Rob and Charlie – they were everything to me. Doing something that lurched us into financial risk wasn't something that sat well.

David had reassured me it would be okay. Luckily he had a good job and would be able to take care of us. I wasn't used to someone taking care of me though. Ever since I was a little girl I'd wanted to stand on my own two feet. I loved working, it gave me a purpose, I didn't want to give that up. I also loved helping people, that's why I became a doctor. My thoughts went back to my patients. I felt a huge pang of guilt for walking away from them.

Guilt, fear, sadness, anger – a cocktail of emotions were turning and churning around in my mind, growing louder and more intrusive in the quiet of the night, until I finally snapped.

I peeled back the duvet, tiptoed across the room and slipped into my thick fleece dressing gown that was hanging from the hook on the back of the door. The cold fabric, chilled by the winter air, sent a shiver down my spine.

David stirred. 'Are you okay?'

'I'm fine, go back to sleep.'

Downstairs, I made myself a cup of warmed milk. I took a seat at our chunky wooden table and stared through the kitchen windows into the night. The infinity of black felt as dark as my future.

I didn't have a formal agreement with my partners about my notice period. We had agreed I would leave the surgery in just three weeks' time.

Leave my surgery – those words stoked my anger again.

I didn't feel it was right! GPs shouldn't be getting paid bonuses for doing their jobs!

I took another furious slurp from my mug.

My partners had also been keen that I keep appointment times to ten minutes, and only address one problem in that time. But often my patients had been waiting weeks to see me, and if they came in with more than one problem I didn't have the heart to tell them they would have to book another appointment, that they would have to wait another three weeks to tell me the rest of what was bothering them. More importantly, one ailment could be related to another; it was important to hear the full story.

I felt more indignant than ever.

I stared through the kitchen window again. But this time I looked past the darkness to see my own reflection.

My hair, short as it was, had managed to find entirely absurd, startled shapes. I flattened it down the best I could with my hand, and swept my fringe from my eyes.

I looked utterly exhausted but I knew I wouldn't be able to get back to sleep until I had got everything off my chest.

I made my way to the study.

I didn't need to switch the light on, the moon was beaming through the large sash windows, illuminating the cluttered room.

The shelves were so packed with medical journals they were warping under the weight, sinking in the middle like a hammock. The desk which overlooked the garden wasn't much better. Either side of the computer were mountains of paperwork. The weight of a life, mountains and mountains of paper, and I was throwing it all away.

Beside the keyboard were silver-framed pictures of my boys in their school uniforms. They sported proud grins. Were they proud of me?

Twenty years. Twenty years of looking after people and it was all over.

I switched on the computer and reached down to turn on the electric heater by my feet. It rattled and hummed, the noise strangely comforting.

I started writing. Pouring my heart out at half past three in the morning, tipping all of my emotions onto the blank page.

It was everything I wished I had expressed in the meeting earlier, every argument against the new contract and their new policies. Explaining exactly how it had forced me into quitting the job I loved.

I wrote for nearly an hour and then sunk back into the padded leather swivel chair, letting out a huge sigh of relief.

What I should have done was pressed 'Save', slipped back under my duvet and snuggled into David, now that I had got everything off my chest.

Instead, I pressed 'Send'.

Chapter Two

I didn't expect to make the front page!

Sitting in my room at the surgery, I found myself staring at my own words, splashed across the pages of *Pulse*, a national magazine for GPs.

'I just ride off into the sunset and no one gives a toss.'

That was what I'd said, but I didn't think they were going to quote me word for word!

I cursed myself for being so impulsive and emotional. What I meant by that line was that I'd worked so hard to try to do a good job, for nearly twenty years, but it felt like it counted for nothing in the end because no one cared. All they wanted to see was boxes being ticked.

I wished I'd packed a pair of sunglasses to hide behind.

But there was nothing I could do about it now. My opinions were in black and white for all to see. The best thing I could do was straighten my back and get on with working out my three weeks' notice at the practice.

I was yo-yoing back and forth between anger and regret again. It wasn't a healthy place to be and thank goodness

I had a half-hour break in my schedule. I grabbed my bag and made a run for some fresh air.

Everywhere I looked I was reminded of what I was losing. As I walked through the waiting room, I could feel dozens of pairs of eyes staring at me in disbelief – the leaving letter I'd written to patients was pinned to the notice board.

I crossed the tree-lined street to the coffee shop opposite the surgery, but the atmosphere in there wasn't much better. Sandra, the pharmacist from the chemist next door, was in front of me in the queue. She'd been dispensing medication as long as I'd been a GP in the area. I thought she was going to mention the article, but she had other news for me.

'It's as if the village is in mourning,' she blurted.

Sandra had become a close friend over the years. She had the kindest face, which was framed by her masses of chestnut hair. She wasn't much over five foot tall, and looked up at me with her dark eyes.

I couldn't respond. I had no idea what to say. She carried on, every word tugging at my heart.

'Your patients are so sad. They don't know what they're going to do without you. Amanda, do you really have to go . . .?'

I gently squeezed Sandra's arm. Really I wanted to throw my arms around her and give her a bear hug.

'I've made my decision, and I'm just going to have to see it through now. I feel terrible though,' I admitted. The urge to cry rose up in me. That was the last thing I needed: to burst into tears in the middle of a coffee shop queue.

Then came the big question. 'But what will you do now?'
Well, yes, what indeed?

'I guess with your experience you could easily get a job
in another practice,' she continued.

That was the last thing I wanted. I'd be faced with the
same problems, just in a different location. But what was I
going to do? I felt like I was going through a bereavement.
I felt sad, lonely, lost, unable to see a way forward, a thick
dark fog of self-doubt and guilt obscuring my vision of the
future.

Suddenly, the roasted aroma of coffee beans smelt acidic,
nauseating and unbearable. The sounds of the café, the
white noise of chatter, the hiss of the milk steamer . . . It
all felt more than I could bear. I felt waves of heat rush up
my neck and I was desperate to return to the chill of the
winter air outside.

It was torture. What had I done?

'I'm going to have to get back to work,' I said to
Sandra.

'But you haven't even had your coffee. We have to do
drinks before you leave . . .' Her voice trailed off as I gave
her the thumbs up and dashed for the door.

Outside, I took a few deep gulps of air, drinking up the
freshness in place of my coffee. I felt like crying. It was all
too much. Seeing my outburst in the magazine, hearing how
my patients were feeling and then, of course, the final panic:
the realisation that I didn't have the faintest idea what I was
going to do with the rest of my life.

Back inside my consultation room, things went from bad to worse when Mr Collins knocked on my door.

If only I could have hidden behind my desk for the afternoon, but there was no getting away.

'Come in,' I said, hiding behind a cheerful voice.

Brian Collins was one of my long-standing patients. He was 56 years of age, tall, with grey receding hair, and was always clean shaven. He had long spindly fingers that always made me think he should play the piano.

Brian poked his head around the door and gingerly made his way across the mottled carpet towards my desk. His steps were uncertain; a man whose confidence had taken several knocks.

He'd been on and off antidepressants for as long as I could remember. They eased his depression, but then he would stop taking them, convinced he was feeling better, only to fall back into a depressive slump.

Brian was typical of so many of the patients I saw at my practice. Wealthy, successful, middle class, well-spoken. The stereotypical pinstripe-suited man who travelled into the city every day. When I'd first started working in the area, he was the type of man I must admit that I felt a bit intimidated by, as I thought they might not trust a young female doctor. But, to my surprise, I managed to win him and many other patients over. I think as much as anything else it was by showing them that I really cared about them. I've always believed that the root cause of many illnesses can be found in the emotional problems that lie bubbling underneath. The problem then became that many of my patients seemed to depend on me as a counsellor, more than as a doctor . . . Mr Collins was no exception.

'What can I do for you, Brian?' I asked, my voice gentle, warm, doing my best to set him at ease.

His eyes were downcast as he slumped into the chair opposite.

'Is it really true you're going?' he said, his eyes filled with worry.

It was the first time I'd come face to face with the effect my departure was having, and it was unbearable. The tension in my little consultation room was palpable.

'Yes, I'm afraid so.'

He fell completely silent for a moment, staring, intently, at one spot on the carpet before finally looking me in the eye. I could see the tears. It was heartbreaking to watch.

He tugged free a tissue from the box on my desk and dabbed the corners of his eyes.

His voice trembled. 'But what will I do without you? You're the only person who understands what I'm going through, and I find it so hard to open up to people.'

His fears were completely natural, and were shared by many people who might feel anxious about changing their doctor.

'Will you be moving to a surgery nearby?'

I opened my mouth to speak, but nothing came out. I was going to tell him no, but the question had thrown me – all the way back into that pit of uncertainty. I swallowed hard and whispered. 'I don't think so.'

His eyes dropped again, crestfallen, and then he suddenly lurched onto his feet.

He shot out his hand, as I imagined he had done hundreds of times in his board meetings, disguising his distress with formality.

'Well, I wish you all the best for the future, Doctor Brown.'

I felt a lump rise in my throat as I shook his hand.

'You've been wonderful and I really appreciate everything you've done for me over the years,' he carried on in his rigid, staccato voice. 'And anyone who has you as their doctor next is blessed.'

I bit my lip – hanging on by a thread to stop myself breaking down in tears. Hiding behind my medicine, I told Mr Collins to continue with the same dose of antidepressants, and to review how he felt in three months.

I walked him to the door and we had a moment's silence, both aware of each other's grief. 'Things will get better,' I encouraged.

With that, he slipped out of the door and I broke down, the avalanche of the day's emotions crashing in on me.

It was no good; a doctor's life is a constant flow of difficult situations, of emotional patients, of pain and sadness and death. I needed to be stronger than that – I *was* stronger than that, always had been – but I just couldn't see how I was going to get through the next few weeks.

My phone rang.

I wanted to leave it ringing, and I almost did, but I needed something – anything – to pull me out of the low mood I was descending into.

'Is that Doctor Brown?' asked a voice on the line.

'Yes, who's speaking?'

'It's Doctor Phil Burn here. I saw your story in *Pulse*.'

My stomach lurched.

'I'm recruiting doctors to work in prisons in the South East of England.'

'Sorry?' I wasn't sure I'd heard correctly.

'I'm looking for a doctor to work in a prison,' he repeated.

I was stunned by the thought. I had been so locked away in my village practice that alternative placements like he was suggesting hadn't really occurred to me.

Dr Burn continued to explain the job. It was a part-time position at a youth prison for 15–18-year-olds, HMP Huntercombe in Oxfordshire, not too far from Henley-On-Thames. 'Would you be interested?' he asked.

The thought of prison conjured up images of fights, stabbing, hangings – the horror often portrayed in films. Could I really see myself working in that world?

On a deeper level, of course, I knew that my immediate mental image of prison life could hardly be accurate. And I needed to do something . . . Something new, something that would challenge me, something that would make all of this feel worthwhile. Something that might help people.

'Yes!' I said, actually shocking myself. I hadn't given

myself time to think deeply, I was relying on gut instinct, I had no idea what the salary was, I should have been asking so many more questions . . .

But how bad could 15–18-year-olds be? My boys, Rob and Charlie, were that age, so hopefully I would be able to relate to the inmates and perhaps they would view me as a mother figure and not a threat.

Had I really been that naïve? Yes. But I would learn.

He went on to explain that not many doctors wanted to work in prisons, as it was seen as an intimidating and unpleasant environment, dealing with difficult, unwilling, unpredictable and possibly violent people.

'But' – and he laughed as he said it – 'anyone as outspoken as you should be able to handle a challenge!'

I couldn't believe it, my candid words in the magazine had opened up a whole new world of possibilities. Dr Burn had recognised the fighting spirit in me.

Just because I was nearing fifty, why shouldn't I try something new? It's never too late to start over. Whether it be your career, your marriage, your lifestyle. That's what I'd been telling my patients for years, and now it was time to embrace the unknown myself.

And maybe I could even make a difference to these boys' lives.

*

Dear God, what have I done?

Back at home, I was questioning my decision. Had I been rash, accepting a job I knew practically nothing about?

I was sitting at the kitchen table doing some background reading into Huntercombe prison.

It was officially classified as a young offenders' institution, having housed teenagers since 2000. It had originally been built as an internment camp during the Second World War and was turned into a prison in 1946.

Unlike adult prisons, which are categorised by letters, from A to D, depending on the seriousness of the crimes of the prisoners locked up, a young offenders' institute has no grade. That didn't reassure me though.

I'm not frightened easily, but I was filled with self-doubt as I read up about the crimes some of these teenagers had committed. It wasn't just theft and burglary but also murder and rape.

I turned to David for advice.

'Do you think I can do it?' I asked

He was peeling the spuds for dinner and laughed. 'Don't be ridiculous, of course you can, you're more than capable.' He smiled. 'You *always* are.'

I loved the fact that he was so supportive of both me and my career. God knows how many evenings he'd spent alone, looking after the boys while I'd worked very long days or been called out in the middle of the night. He understood my drive and my need to help others. He understood I had worked too hard for my career to give it up.

'I'm going to be treating teenagers who have committed some very serious crimes!'

It was hard to comprehend that boys my sons' age could have killed someone, raped someone, abused a young child.

'But they need a doctor, too. And I can't think of a better person for the job,' David said.

He was right. I wasn't there to judge; my job was to try to make people better.

'But it's a prison. Have I got the guts to handle it?'

I heard the plop of another peeled potato being dropped into the saucepan of water, then David turned around and looked me in the eye.

'Do I have to remind you of some of the brave things you've done in the past? Do you remember that bloke who had a knife to his throat . . .?'

Chapter Three

It was a scorching summer's day and I was sipping on an ice cold drink and having a quick bite to eat at my desk in my lunch break.

A gentle breeze lifted the curtains as it blew into my consultation room, tickling the back of my neck.

I battled to keep my eyes open; in that heat I could easily have dozed off for a few minutes. Suddenly the peace was broken by screaming and the sound of footsteps hurtling down the corridor.

My door burst wide open. One of my patients, Jenny Scott, was standing in front of me, breathless, panic stricken.

'Amanda, you have to come with me now,' she screeched.

Her normally perfectly styled hair was windswept and tangled. Her usual composure was shattered.

'It's Jonathan – he's got a knife and he says he's going to kill himself. I don't know what to do. He's at home . . . please come.'

Jonathan was Jenny's husband, an alcoholic who suffered from severe mood swings. I'd been treating both of them for years. Without a second thought, I grabbed my bag, filled with all the equipment and medicines I carry to my home visits, and chased after her into the surgery car park.

She sped off in her car, but I knew exactly where to go. I'd been to their house on many home visits in the past.

It was less than five minutes from the surgery, in a pretty lane with beautiful houses on either side. Large homes, with large gardens and expensive cars parked in the driveways. Many people would look at the area and think that the people who lived there surely had to be happy. But, from my experience, inside many of those magnificent houses, behind the seemingly perfect façades, there lurked a lot of anguish and unhappiness. A significant proportion of the medical problems I treated were brought on by stress and financial pressures. I learned early on in my career that money very often doesn't buy happiness

Turning into their road, the dappled sunlight trickling through the trees was replaced with the blue and white flashing lights of several police cars. They were parked outside the Scotts' home. Half a dozen armed police officers wearing protective vests surrounded the house. I parked and got out of my car. What had I walked into? It looked like a hostage negotiation scene from a film.

Jenny was standing behind one of the police cars. She beckoned me over. A police officer stepped into my path, his hand outstretched, ready to stop me.

'It's okay, I'm his doctor,' I explained.

The police officer moved aside and Jenny ran forward, a look of relief washing across her face.

'Thank God you're here, Amanda.'

Her whole body was trembling, but she wasn't crying. Jenny was a tough, resilient woman, and could cope with a great deal. Goodness knows she'd had to over the years. It wasn't uncommon for Jonathan to lose his temper, but I never thought I'd see the day when police cars were parked outside their house.

'So, what's happened?' I asked.

'I don't know, I don't understand, one minute he was fine and the next . . .' Jenny paused to compose herself. 'We were having lunch together. I got up to get the salad cream out of the fridge and noticed three of the wine bottles were missing. Three!

'I know he likes to drink, Amanda, but three bottles by lunch was a lot even by his standards. I was tired, I was angry, and I asked him where they had gone.'

Her voice started to tremble and, knowing Jenny, she was blaming herself for whatever happened next.

'He started shouting that I shouldn't have asked him, and the next thing I knew he'd pulled the carving knife out of the drawer and was holding it against his neck. He was telling me he didn't deserve me, and he was going to kill himself.'

She looked to me for reassurance. 'This is my fault, isn't it?'

I squeezed her arm. 'No, Jenny,' I stressed, not for the first time. 'This is not your fault.'

I felt deeply sorry for her. I couldn't imagine what she had suffered over the years. And being the strong, independent woman that she was, I imagine she had kept a lot of her pain locked up inside. I also felt deeply sorry for Jonathan, living with anxiety and depression, turning to alcohol to numb his pain.

'I tried to get him to put down the knife,' she said. 'But that only made him hold it closer to his neck. I was terrified, so I ran. He listens to you, Amanda, please will you talk to him?'

I felt the pressure building.

I turned to one of the police officers and asked if they had approached Jonathan.

'Not yet. We have to wait for legal authority to enter. Won't take long but right now . . .' He shrugged. 'Well, we're stuck here.'

'What about me?' I asked. 'Can I go in?'

'Legally? Yes, you're his doctor, and have reason to assume he may be hurt.' He looked at me and the fear in his eyes, the concern for my safety, nearly changed my mind. 'You shouldn't, though. You should wait for us to get clearance and then we'll all go in together.'

But that was no good, was it? Jonathan needed me. Jenny needed me. It was my job to help and I was obliged to carry out my duties.

I walked up the driveway.

The Scotts' house was very beautiful, with a large weeping willow in the middle of the lawn, and flowerbeds filled with stunning roses and brightly coloured summer flowers. Rectangular flowerboxes hung along the wall by the front door, and flowerpots filled with pansies and lavender lined the driveway.

My heart pounded as I drew closer to the porch. I was nervous about what to expect on the other side of the door. There was a chance Jonathan could turn the knife on me.

It felt like one of the longest walks of my life. I turned back to see everyone's eyes watching me. Jenny's hand was clutched over her mouth and the police officers were poised, their hands hovering over their weapons, ready to jump in at any moment.

I took one last look back and then plunged in.

The front door was ajar. I pushed it open with my fingertips, stepping into the hallway. The house was eerily quiet, my shoes sounding far too loud on the wooden floor.

I called out. 'Jonathan?'

Silence.

'Jonathan, it's Doctor Brown.'

There was still no reply but I kept moving, into the kitchen, bracing myself for what I was about to see.

But he wasn't in the kitchen any more.

I called out, again. 'Jonathan? It's Doctor Brown. I've come to see if you're okay.'

I heard a noise coming from the living room.

The nervousness I'd felt had left me now. I needed to find him as quickly as possible. I moved into the living room.

'Oh, Jonathan!' I gasped as I turned the corner.

He was standing in front of their leather sofa, his slim frame outlined by the sun streaming through the skylights. The knife, pressed hard against his throat, was glinting. He was swaying slightly, drunk, a sweat glistening on his forehead, his lips wet.

He stared at me, not saying a word.

I was shocked. I knew him well, as he had confided in me over the years about his problems, and I'd come to regard him more as a friend than a patient. My heart went out to him that he felt so desperate he wanted to kill himself.

His lips were white, his face drained of colour. His eyes were agitated, his whole body tense. But still he didn't speak; he just kept the knife clamped to his throat.

I didn't have any choice but to try to take it from him.

I started to gently walk towards him. My voice was soft as I said, 'Please, please, Jonathan, give me the knife.'

He was frozen to the spot.

'Let me have the knife, it's going to be fine.'

Still no reply, as I softly, slowly moved forward. What was going through his mind? Was he about to cut his own throat? Was he about to turn the knife on me?

The sound of police radios and talking were coming from outside the window.

I couldn't see any lacerations on his neck, but the tip of the knife was pressing hard against his skin. Any trigger could set him off.

'Jonathan—' I started, but didn't finish my sentence. Suddenly, he lurched towards me, the knife in his right hand.

It all happened so quickly. I froze, suddenly certain that I'd made a terrible mistake, that I was going to die, there in that opulent living room. Blood spilling onto a carpet few could afford. I'd gone there to help but Jonathan was too far gone, too lost to see clearly. His arms stretching out towards me, the knife shining, looking sharp enough to cut a slit in the air itself.

Yes. I was about to die.

He flung his arms around my neck and flopped onto my shoulders, letting go of his grasp of the large carving knife. It made a small *thunk* as it dropped onto the living room floor behind me. Part of my brain heard it fall, recognised that the danger was past; the rest of me was occupied with the sobbing Jonathan. I stood there, holding him up, as he sobbed and sobbed and sobbed.

'It's going to be okay,' I said, stroking his back as I would a child who desperately needed a hug and reassurance.

When his breathing had calmed a little I told him we needed to go outside, that Jenny was waiting for him.

His voice was thick with tears. 'How can she ever forgive me?'

'She loves you, we all care about you. Jenny would be distraught if anything happened to you,' I said.

I led him out of the living room and towards the front door.

He was wobbling still, drunk and disorientated, and I propped him up as we walked into the sunshine together.

I was relieved to see the flashing lights of an ambulance.

'I want you to go to the hospital for me,' I said. 'They'll help. Can you do that for me?'

He nodded.

Jenny ran towards us, taking her sobbing husband into her arms. I was so thankful that he was safe. I looked at the two of them, unable to shake the thought that one – or both – of them could have died today if things had gone differently. Ultimately, while I may have helped to ground him, Jonathan had held on to enough strength – just enough – to stop himself from doing something that would have torn their lives apart.

I stood back as the paramedics helped him into the ambulance, to take him to the psychiatric ward of the local hospital. Jenny followed in her car. He was in need of expert help, more help than I could give him.

I watched as they disappeared from view and then got back into my car and drove slowly back to work. I had other patients to see.

Chapter Four

I remembered those nerve-racking steps towards Jonathan and Jenny's house, as I walked towards the entrance of HMP Huntercombe. My heart was pounding just as much, my palms moist with anticipation as to what was around the corner.

And then suddenly, just as it had all those years ago, courage kicked in.

I straightened my back and walked on with confidence and purpose.

It was daunting but exciting. I was reinventing myself.

My thoughts were broken by the noise of a large white van rolling up to the prison gates. It had the distinctive tiny blacked-out windows running along the sides, the ones the paparazzi try to reach their cameras up to when high-profile prisoners leave court. I wondered who was inside it.

As the huge metal gates opened, I was able to get a brief glimpse of what lay on the other side. A concrete yard, some more fencing, half a dozen prison officers . . . and then it all vanished from view as the gates slammed shut.

The intimidating façade of the prison wall, with its barbed wire twisting over the top, was a stark reminder of what life held in store for those being dropped off.

I arrived at the gatehouse, where a thick glass screen separated me from the officers who kept a close eye on the monitors to see who was coming and going.

It was like being at passport control at the airport, slowly being given the once-over.

'What's your name?' asked a small stocky man with a thick Essex accent.

'Doctor Amanda Brown,' I replied, loudly, just in case he might not hear me through the thick glass screen.

'Have you got your ID with you?'

I pulled out my passport and driver's licence from my bag, and passed them through the hatch that he clicked open.

There was a long pause as he checked my ID, and then I heard the rumble of a big heavy metal door sliding open.

I stepped forward, taking another half-step to make sure the monstrous door didn't clip me as it closed.

I was now on the other side, standing in a narrow corridor. An officer spoke through another glass screen, and told me that someone from Healthcare would come along soon to meet me. I moved along the corridor slightly, to a small room lined from floor to ceiling with lockers. This, presumably, would be where my belongings would be stored, the things I could take inside being limited for safety reasons.

Straightaway, a reminder of what I was facing: a job where the contents of my pockets could get someone killed unless I was careful.

The head of Healthcare arrived, greeting me with a friendly smile and a handshake. I hadn't seen Dawn Kendall since my interview, six months previously – the process of getting security clearance and having contracts drawn up for the job had taken that long.

She had a clipboard in one hand and a large set of keys in the other, which clinked as she rolled them between her fingers. She looked like she meant business, with her black trouser suit and white blouse.

I was given a locker in which to store my phone, bag and coat, then she unlocked another large solid metal door, and I followed her through. That was locked behind us, the sound heavy and horribly final. A large metal gate followed; again keys jangled, locks turned. Then – finally – we were in the prison grounds.

'Once you have your key training you'll be able to do this yourself.'

She turned around and grinned at me. 'But for now, you're stuck with me escorting you.'

I'd liked Dawn from the moment I met her. She was a large lady with a big personality to match. I got the sense she wanted to mother the boys because, somewhere, deep down, I'm sure she felt sorry for them.

I believed that most of the staff genuinely wanted to make a difference, and I hoped I was also going to be able to.

We walked across the courtyard, then through another metal door and another gate, and finally we were in the Healthcare department of the prison.

The walls were brightly coloured and there were a variety of drawings and paintings stuck on them. 'All done by the boys,' Dawn proudly announced.

She walked briskly ahead, filling me in on some facts that belied the innocent-looking appearance of the place.

'Huntercombe is home to 360 of the country's most troubled teenagers. Sadly, many of the kids inside here have come from troubled families. Violence is all they've known.'

We turned a corner and I skipped to keep up.

'The UK has the most juveniles locked up behind bars in Europe. This age group, 15–18-year-olds, has the worst reoffending rate of all: 82 percent are likely to commit another crime within two years of being released.

'You're not shocked easily are you, Amanda?' she asked as she unlocked the door to the clinical room.

I shook my head.

'Good, because these boys can be rude, they can be aggressive, particularly when they don't get the medication they want.

'Some of them will have had drug addictions, and will want you to prescribe them strong painkillers and sleeping pills. These need to be avoided at all costs; they're highly addictive and can sometimes be used as currency, to trade for cigarettes or items of clothing. Some of the boys can also be bullied, attacked for them. Drugs are a commodity here; we need to be careful.'

In the twenty years I'd worked as a GP I'd only looked after one patient who was addicted to any medication. My experience wasn't going to be much use to me. I had so much to learn.

The Healthcare department was where the prison GPs ran their clinics, alongside other healthcare professionals, including the dentist, psychiatrist, optician and GUM consultant – a doctor specialising in sexual health.

Dawn informed me that there were a lot of self-harmers in Huntercombe, and to prepare myself for seeing some horrific scars and shocking wounds.

She sighed. 'It's very sad, but often it's an outlet for these boys. They are lonely, depressed, some just want to die. They turn to self-harming as a way of offsetting the pain and stress they're feeling inside their heads.

'A lot of these lads don't want anyone to see their wounds, or the scars from cigarette burns, the scalds made with boiling water.'

I felt a huge pang of pity. It was awful to think boys the same age as my sons felt so desperate and helpless that they needed to self-harm in such a way. No one should suffer like that.

Again, I hadn't seen many patients who self-harmed while I worked at my surgery. More to learn.

I wouldn't be dealing directly with mental-health issues; they would be handled by the psychiatrist. However, I might have to tend to their wounds, particularly if they had become infected and needed antibiotics. I might also have to re-prescribe antidepressants if the psychiatrist wasn't in.

I had been expecting to deal with the common complaints that teenagers usually present with, such as acne, asthma, skin infections and rashes, etc – conditions I'd seen hundreds of times over the years in my old practice. But now the type of patient would be very different.

A couple of nurses were popping in and out of rooms along the corridor, and Dawn called them over to introduce me. I was given a lovely warm welcome by both.

'The turnover rate of doctors is high in prisons,' Dawn explained, 'so everyone is hoping you'll stay with us. We need some consistency here.

'Apparently, working with the 18-to-21 age group can be the most challenging of all. They're the most notori-ously difficult. Too much testosterone in too confined an area. They're always fighting, with each other mostly, but sometimes with the prison officers as well.

'That's why I like working here.' She stopped outside a pale green painted door. 'Despite the government statistics on reoffenders, I feel like we still have a chance with boys this age, to help put them on the right path in life.'

Dawn unlocked the door and pushed it open.

'And this is where you will be working.' She stood back to let me pass.

It was a far cry from what I was used to, but it wasn't as bad as I had expected. It was small, clean, and had the essentials. There was a desk and shelves, all compact and well designed, as if it had come straight out of IKEA. There was also an examination couch on the other side of the room, with blue tissue paper placed on top, ready for my first patient.

The lovely thing about the little room though, was that there was a window – even if there were big metal bars in front of it! I wasn't expecting to have natural sunlight, so although the view wasn't up to much I was grateful. I peered out on to the tarmac yard outside.

'Can get a bit noisy when the boys are walking across the yard,' said Dawn. 'Silence is a luxury in this place!'

She was standing on the opposite side of the room, stroking her top lip with her forefinger as she tried to remember any details she may have forgotten. I had so many questions but I decided it was better to just get on with the job and save them for later. It seemed to me that this was the kind of place that you learn as you go along; sink or swim.

'A nurse will run the clinic with you, she will let the boys in and out and tend to all the minor things through there.' Dawn pointed to an adjoining room.

'Ah speak of the devil.' Dawn took a step backwards to make way for a petite, pretty lady, in her early sixties, wearing blue trousers and a long blue tunic top. A biro was peeping out of the top of her breast pocket.

She may have been five foot nothing, but I could tell I wouldn't want to get on her wrong side. Nobody would. She had an authoritative air about her.

Dawn introduced her.

'Amanda, this is Wendy – or Matron, as the boys like to call her.'

Wendy stared up at me through her thick dark fringe. She had a blunt bob cut which was striped with grey hairs. Her face was stern, but she had kind eyes.

'Wendy must be one of our longest-serving staff. Thirty years now.'

'Thirty-two next May,' Wendy corrected her, as she busied about doing her things, darting in and out of the room.

'If you have any questions, she'll be able to help you.'

Just as Dawn was leaving, she spun around and looked me straight in the eye. Her voice was hard now.

'One last thing. Make sure you do not reveal anything personal about yourself to the boys. Keep where you live, any details of your family, private.'

The words were chilling.

I nodded obediently.

'It's not permitted for any prison or medical staff to have any sort of communication with inmates after their release.'

I nodded again. Things suddenly seemed to get a lot more serious. I'd been so used to being entwined in my patients' lives at the surgery. I had followed their journeys over the years, visited them at their homes, watched their lives evolve. This was a completely different way of approaching medicine. I would be seeing prisoners in my clinic who I might never see again.

Dawn softened as she saw my flash of concern. 'You'll be fine. It'll be a challenge.'

With that, she disappeared along the corridor.

*

My thoughts were interrupted by a thud on my desk. I looked up to see Wendy had given me a large plastic box of files. Inside were orange A4 folders, of varying thickness, each marked with a number – the prison number of the boys I would be seeing that morning. It was wrong to make the assumption that the thicker files would be the more demanding patients, but from everything I'd heard that morning, I couldn't help but jump to that conclusion.

'Doesn't make for light reading,' Wendy grimaced. 'And here's the list of boys you will be seeing.' She placed a sheet of paper on the desk.

'Thank you,' I smiled, grateful for her help. I knew I could do with having Wendy on my side.

She carried on whizzing back and forth between rooms, making the final preparations. I glanced at my watch.

'What happens now?' I asked, as she reappeared.

Wendy explained that the officers from the various wings were collecting the boys, who had either put in a request to see me, or who one of the nurses had decided needed to be seen.

'They then wait in the communal area until I call them in,' she explained.

I peered out of the door to look at the waiting area, which had approximately twenty plastic chairs set out in neat rows.

'Everything is plastic here,' Wendy explained. 'From the chairs to the cutlery.'

'Oh?'

'To try to prevent them from self-harming,' she said.

And again, I was forced to face the reality that some of these young people felt so desperate that harming themselves seemed the only escape.

'You'd better get set up, they'll be arriving any minute.' Wendy nodded, and left the office again.

I returned to my desk and glanced over the names of the boys I was about to see. What had they done? I couldn't know about their crimes, that was a detail not recorded on their medical notes. Besides, I would have hoped that knowing about the severity of their crimes wouldn't have affected my ability to help them. Yes, I would hope that ... but it was a relief not to have to prove as much. Who were they? What were they coming to see me for? Of course, it was no different to any new patient, not really ...

By the time I'd read to the end of the list, the noise from the waiting room had swelled into loud chatter and raucous laughter.

An authoritative voice bellowed, 'Oi, keep it down in here!' That must have been the prison officer in the waiting room.

Which only led to more sniggers.

And to the prison officer becoming even more irate.

'Keep it down in here, I said!' he shouted, banging his fist on the door.

'Ah, you can fuck off an' all!' came the reply.

Then, in a flash, chairs were screeching across the floor, more shouting, more swearing, scuffling, threats, then silence.

I nearly jumped out of my skin when Wendy knocked on my door.

'That's what happens if you put a bunch of rowdy teenagers in a small room together,' she said, poking her head inside and rolling her eyes. 'I've got Jerome Scott here.'

I pulled Jerome's file from the plastic box. It was as thick as a book.

'Come in!' I called out.

I prepared myself to meet my first patient in prison.

Chapter Five

Jerome was tall, skinny, and wore his grey prison tracksuit bottoms low enough to show off his boxer shorts. He was pale, spotty and had a diamanté stud in both ears. His hair was shaved along the sides and spiked with gel on top. He looked like every other teenager who had spent too many hours indoors playing video games.

It was only his eyes that told a different story. They were bloodshot, puffy, hollowed out by the shadowy purple circles underneath. He looked as if he hadn't slept in months, and I prepared myself for his request for sleeping tablets.

'Come on in, take a seat.' I welcomed the teenager in the usual friendly manner I'd always greeted my patients with, in my old surgery.

Jerome swaggered across the room and slumped into the chair opposite. He automatically slipped into a slouch with his left leg outstretched and his right elbow hooked over the top of the chair.

'How can I help you?' I asked, leafing through his most recent medical notes to familiarise myself. Antidepressants, medication for anxiety. Bruising to ribs and left cheek and

cuts to forehead, following a fight with his cellmate. I looked
up to check how well the wounds on his face had healed.

'It's my feet, Miss.'

I was taken aback a little. After such a build-up, and a
complex history, I wasn't expecting such a seemingly minor
complaint.

'Oh dear. What's wrong with your feet?'

'They hurt when I walk. It's these shoes, innit.'

Jerome lifted one of his black trainers into the air, which
I assumed must be part of the prison uniform. He then
returned to his slouch and started biting his nails, or the
little bits of nail he had left. I noticed a tattoo of a snake
wrapped around a sword on his left wrist, the tip of the
blade peeping out from under the cuff of his jumper.

'What sort of pain are you feeling, and whereabouts on
your feet?' I could believe those shoes weren't the most
comfortable.

'I've got blisters everywhere, Miss. I can barely walk, it's
so painful. I can't be doing with these trainers.'

It was strange to be called Miss, but I suppose Jerome
saw me as an authoritative figure, like a teacher – unlike
my previous patients who, on the whole, had viewed me
as a friend. Did I want that responsibility? Could I take it?

I moved around to the other side of the desk to take a
closer look, asking Jerome to remove his socks and shoes.
He waved his slightly smelly bare foot in the air to reveal
the tiniest of blisters on his right heel.

His eyes looked sheepishly to the ground.

'It's killing me. I can barely walk!'

He didn't seem to have any problems swaggering into my office a moment ago, I thought. I started to wonder if there was a bit more to his complaint.

'Why don't you pop next door, and the nurse can give you some plasters for your blisters.'

The words had barely left my mouth when Jerome fired back with his own diagnosis and cure.

'Can you just write me a note saying I can wear my own trainers? That way I won't get blisters no more.'

I suddenly cottoned on to what was going on. There must be some sort of loophole whereby the prisoners could wear their own shoes on medical grounds. Whether the trainers would be sent in by his family, I didn't know, but I was pretty sure that's what Jerome was after.

It was my first day on the job and I needed to be careful not to break any rules.

Turning a little firmer with my tone, I suggested, 'Let's try out the plasters first and see how that goes.'

Jerome huffed loudly.

'But Miss,' he whined.

He sat there for a moment, sulking, waiting for me to come around to his way of thinking. Nibbling on his nails.

I thought about what I would say to my boys if they were trying to get their way.

I smiled and explained it was my first day in the prison and that he needed to use the plasters first, but I promised I would find out the rules and regulations surrounding the boys wearing their own trainers instead of prison-issue shoes.

After more huffing and puffing Jerome reluctantly agreed to try the plasters, and as he walked off to see Wendy in the next room he turned back and flashed me a mischievous grin.

'See you next week then, Miss.'

*

The rest of my morning surgery was a succession of minor ailments, with at least three more trainer requests, all with similarly feeble excuses.

Two of the boys complained of achy feet, the other of painful toenails. It seemed ludicrous that a doctor's time was taken up by dealing with kids wanting their own footwear. It was something I would have to take up with Dawn, but first I needed to tell Wendy about the massive faux pas I'd made with one of the other boys.

'I told him I liked the orange jumpsuit he was wearing. That it was a bit more bright and colourful than the grey tracksuit. He said "Thanks, Miss, I get to wear orange because I tried to escape!"'

Wendy howled with laughter.

'I suppose he won't be making a run for it again in that jumpsuit. He'll stick out like a sore thumb!' I laughed along with her.

For a moment I looked at the severe Wendy, and she

looked at me, and I felt reassured. Yes, we were going to get along just fine.

It was funny, but it was also strange to think that someone I was treating for something as routine as a minor ear infection had tried to break out of a high-security prison, maybe hours earlier. I was dealing with the ordinary in what was otherwise an extraordinary foreign world.

I turned to Wendy and asked, 'So what's with these boys wanting trainers?'

If anyone would know what tricks the boys were up to, Wendy would.

She chuckled. 'It's not "cool" to wear prison shoes, and they'll do anything to try and wear their own trainers. It allows them to maintain some sort of identity in here.'

Wendy looked me in the eye. 'You've just got to be firm with them, or they'll run rings around you.'

I'd worked that out pretty quickly. If I gave into one, they would all be queuing up – kids demanding trainers all week long.

'These boys are crafty. If they see you're a soft touch, they'll immediately take advantage,' she warned me. 'They're constantly testing you, pushing you to the limit. Like most teenagers. But don't forget some of them are very experienced at lying and manipulating. It's easy to forget they're in here because they've committed a crime.'

Wendy was right. It was easy to blot out the fact that the boys were criminals, when I was treating them for very run-of-the-mill medical problems. Apart from their bad language, on the whole, they seemed quite well-behaved.

After three weeks in Huntercombe, apart from getting thoroughly irritated by the trainer requests, I realised I was having an invigorating time in my new world. It was different and challenging and I felt like I'd been given a new lease of life. The cloud that had hung over me when I left my practice was rapidly lifting. I was beginning to feel accepted and to enjoy feeling worthwhile again. Might I even be making a difference?

I was living in a bit of a bubble in the Healthcare department. I knew little about the other areas of the prison, what went on in the wings, even what the cells looked like. I knew nothing about the boys outside the fifteen-minute consultations they had with me. I'd only run into the governor once or twice. I was in and out, twice a week, now with my own set of keys, treating seemingly ordinary spotty teenagers, with ordinary medical complaints. I was even liking my new name: Miss.

But as with every bubble, it had to burst at some point. And Wendy's words of warning came true sooner than expected.

I blamed the waiting-room system. There was a high likelihood that putting a lot of teenage boys together in a confined space could lead to trouble.

My Wednesday-morning surgery had started like all the others so far. A big pile of files on my desk, and a list of the boys I would be seeing over the next few hours.

As usual, I had no idea beforehand of what they were coming in for.

I knew they were a rowdy lot, though, as there had been a great deal more laughter and shouting coming from the waiting area than usual. The prison officer had screamed at them to shut up a number of times, but I was too far away to hear what they had been saying, other than a load of effing and blinding.

When Wendy knocked on my door, her face said a thousand words. Her mouth twisted into a grimace as she wished me luck.

'Thanks, Wen,' I said, before taking a large sip of coffee from my mug. A caffeine hit before I started my clinic.

There were only nine boys on the list that day, and the first one, Danny Farr, had been to see a doctor three weeks ago about his feet. *Three guesses what he's come back for*, I thought, as the 17-year-old made his way into my room.

Short, stocky, and wearing his own clothes, Danny sank down into the chair opposite me. He had strikingly chiselled features, with high cheekbones and a shaved head. His legs were spread wide apart, his arms dangling by his side as he assumed a relaxed pose.

I started things off.

'Morning, Danny, how are you today?'

'I'm okay, Miss.' He coughed loudly. 'Apart from, I got this problem.'

'Go on?' I encouraged him.

'Well, it's a bit embarrassing, Miss.'

I smiled, trying to put him at ease. I knew boys could feel awkward confiding in a woman. 'Don't worry, there's nothing I haven't seen or heard before.'

'It's my . . .' he dropped his gaze to his crotch. 'I think I've got a . . . a spot on my . . .'

'Penis?' I finished off his sentence to speed up the guessing game.

It wasn't really my job as a GP to deal with sexual health, that was left to the 'Dick Doctor' – as the boys called him – the doctor who ran the GUM, or genitourinary medicine clinic. But of course I would have a look if they needed me to.

He looked bashful. 'Yes, Miss.'

'Okay, would you like me to have a look to check it for you?' I said, trying to spare his embarrassment.

He dropped his boxers. At first glance I couldn't see the spot, and we had a good look for it, just to reassure him, but it wasn't there.

As he zipped up his jeans, Danny grinned, showing his crooked teeth. 'I could of sworn I saw it. I thought I'd caught some disease or something.'

'No, you're fine, but you can put your name down for the GUM clinic if you find any more spots or blisters,' I said as he disappeared out the door.

Two minutes later I had Dave Samuel sitting in my consultation room, with surprisingly much the same complaint.

'Got a lump on my balls and I'm scared I've got cancer,' the teenager confessed.

At that moment I heard an eruption of laughter from the waiting room, fading into the corridor. I thought I saw a smirk creep across Dave's face, but if one had, it was gone seconds later.

'Well, we'd better have a look then,' I told him steadily.

Dave stood up, towering over me. He had the same pasty, blotchy skin as most of the teenagers I'd seen, and a scruffy bit of stubble on his face.

I asked him to lie on the couch so that I could examine him. Wendy was busy in the adjoining room so could not chaperone me in the clinic that day.

I pulled the screen around the couch and with his consent I examined his scrotum, and found no lumps or anything abnormal.

Another thunderclap of laughter exploded next door, sending Dave into a fit of giggles.

'Sorry, Doc, I laugh when I get embarrassed.' He stifled his sniggers with his fist.

'You're fine, you can get dressed.'

'What a relief. Thanks, Miss,' Dave said, then quickly scuttled out of my room.

I sighed. What a morning.

I took another sip, of my now lukewarm coffee. Wendy popped her head around the door for a quick moan about how noisy the boys were being.

'I can't think why they're making such a racket,' she hissed. 'There's a new PO on duty and he hasn't taken them in hand. I'll do it myself if he doesn't.'

Wendy was feisty, I didn't doubt her for a second.

'I'll send in the next lad,' she said.

The next boy complained of exactly the same thing, a lump in his scrotum. I examined him and found nothing abnormal, and on it went. Every boy in my surgery that morning came in complaining of something wrong with his genitals.

Of course I had twigged that something was up, so to speak, by the time the fifth lad walked into my surgery with an erection holding up his tracksuit bottoms like a tent pole.

He was tall, well-built and oozing confidence. His tracksuit bottoms were hanging around his backside, and a wry smile curled across his mouth. He swaggered towards me and dropped his trousers and boxers and practically plonked his erection on my desk.

'Is it big enough miss?' he smirked.

A rush of anger came over me. I was furious at his attempt to intimidate me. How dare they come into my office and try to abuse me? Wasn't I doing everything I could to help them? I cared! I wanted to make things better, and all they could do was this? A male doctor wouldn't have had this problem.

I didn't – couldn't – show I was fazed by it, though, as that would have given him the satisfaction he was hoping for. I'd mastered a poker face over my years as a GP, perfecting an ability to hide shock – mostly so I could put people at ease, but in this case, to put someone in his place.

I shrugged.

'It seems pretty normal to me,' I said dismissively, and then got rid of him pretty sharpish. He was just trying to wind me up and I had no time for it.

There was another eruption of laughter as he walked back to the waiting room, no doubt getting a high five from all the boys. The clamour eventually died down as the prison officers took the teenagers back to their wings, while I sat there, raging.

I couldn't wait to vent my anger to Wendy.

'What was that all about?' I exploded. I told her about the boy with an erection and she was shocked and appalled.

She shook her head in dismay. 'That shouldn't have happened, Amanda.'

'Seeing their dicks isn't a big deal to me, I've seen hundreds over the years, but I don't like people trying to intimidate me,' I said, still angry.

It was horrible to think that boys the same age as my sons could act in such a threatening manner. But in a way I was glad; their behaviour had removed any illusions. These were not just any teenagers, these were not just any patients.

'I totally agree. I'm going to report this to Dawn, don't you worry about that,' Wendy said, her hands on her hips. 'I thought there was a lot of whispering and laughter going on in the waiting room. They must have hatched a plan when they arrived. That's the problem with putting them all together. They're bored, looking to make mischief.'

'Testing me to see if I will break,' I said. 'Well, I won't.'

*

I was glad to have David to offload on to that evening. As usual, he was his calm, rational self. He listened as I ranted about the boys, and then reminded me I didn't have to carry on if I wasn't enjoying the job.

He turned the sports channel on mute as I kicked off my shoes and threw myself back into the sofa.

'I can't run away from a job because they try to wind me up one day. It's a fact of life that sometimes you have to deal with things that are insulting and degrading.'

'You don't have to convince me,' David said.

'I mean, I'm incredibly privileged to see a world most people wouldn't have a clue about,' I continued.

'As I said, you don't have to convince me.'

I sunk a bit further into the worn folds of the leather, lifting my feet onto the footstool. I closed my eyes. Maybe David had a point. I was trying to convince someone: myself.

I was enjoying my new job. I was certain I was on the right career path, but something was niggling at me. I hadn't found meaning in what I was doing. Was I making any difference to these boys' lives, other than a quick patch-up job? Could anyone make a difference, or were they too guarded, their walls of self-defence as high and impenetrable as those of the prison?

My limbs grew heavier, and before long I was dozing. Not even the cheers and chanting from the rugby fans on the television could wake me.

Chapter Six

Jared Keane wasn't like all the other boys I'd seen at Huntercombe.

For a long time, I'd been hoping for something more rewarding from my work, and the breakthrough came with an 18-year-old who was months from being transferred to a prison for 18-to-21 year olds.

As soon as he walked into my surgery, I knew there was more to his seemingly simple complaint of back pain.

By now I'd treated countless cases of back problems. These were mostly caused by the paper-thin mattresses and rock-hard beds, or by overdoing weightlifting in the gym.

Jared was shy, unassuming, and avoided eye contact, which was a shame because he had beautiful dark eyes and a very sweet smile. He had the typical buzz-cut hairstyle and bad skin. He had characters tattooed across his knuckles, and a dozen superficial lacerations sliced across both wrists. They were equally spaced, the product of time and precision. From his notes I could see he had used a plastic yoghurt pot as a tool to slice himself.

Jared caught me looking at his self-harm wounds and

pulled his grey jumper sleeves over his wrists, nervously tugging at the fabric.

The cuts were fresh but not infected, and he was due to see the psychiatrist later on in the day to review his mental-health issues.

Anyone who self-harmed in prison was on an ACCT book (Assessment Care in Custody and Teamwork). It's a document that helps to ensure their safety, with repeated observations and entries by the members of staff who know them, commenting on their presentation and mood. If anyone was suspected of being at high risk of suicide, they were observed twenty-four hours a day in a gated cell.

I tried to put Jared at ease by asking him about the history of his back pain, hoping it might open the door to learning a little more about him.

I've always believed that in order to fully comprehend what's going on with someone's health, you have to try to understand them as a person. With Jared, there was clearly a lot going on underneath the surface.

People self-harm for many reasons, but mostly it's to displace the pain they feel in their minds. It can be anything from a scratch on a wrist to attempted suicide. When I had first arrived at Huntercombe, I'd been shocked by how common it was amongst the boys, but over time I'd come to understand why. The loneliness, the overwhelming sense of helplessness and hopelessness, the intense feeling of claustrophobia from being locked up.

Guilt was also a big contributor. Some of these boys had

committed terrible crimes, and were struggling to live with themselves. Others felt guilty for letting a loved one or a family member down.

As with all the other boys I had seen, I had no idea what Jared was inside for, and I didn't feel it was my place to ask. If he wanted to tell me, that was up to him.

He rubbed the lower left side of his back. 'I've been having these pains in my lower back ever since I've been here,' he said.

'How long is that, Jared?'

'Too long, Miss.' He sighed deeply, pushing the air out through his pursed lips. 'Two and a half years. And I got another three to do yet.'

'You're moving?'

'That's right, Miss.'

It must have been a relatively serious crime to warrant a five-and-half-year sentence. Perhaps armed robbery. It was hard to know.

I wanted to look at his back with him standing up, so asked him to roll up his sweatshirt. He was reluctant, and I soon found out why.

His lower back was riddled with old scars from cigarette burns. They looked like small craters dotted across his skin. It was hard to see how he could have done it to himself. I immediately suspected those cigarettes had been stubbed out by someone else.

He was clearly uncomfortable with being so exposed, so I rolled his jumper back down and felt his back through the fabric.

'Ow!' he yelped, as I touched his left side.

I apologised, pressing all over the area to make sure the pain was localised to that one spot. It was, and I was certain it was muscular pain, most likely caused by his mattress, or lack of a decent one.

I then asked him to lie on the couch so that I could examine him further.

'I've been trying to lie on my other side at night, but that hasn't helped my sleep much. I can't sleep as it is, and now I feel like I'm in some sort of straitjacket because I can't move either.'

'It can't be nice sleeping on those beds,' I said sympathetically.

He caught me looking at his wrists and jumped in before I could ask.

'I'm fine, you don't need to look at them,' he snapped. His voice hoarse with emotion.

I softened my tone, my gaze.

'Okay, I won't do anything you don't feel happy with, Jared. Why don't you come and take a seat again?'

As he slumped back into the chair opposite, I wrote a prescription for painkillers on his medication chart, avoiding anything too strong or with a potential for addiction.

As I signed it off, I tried to delve a little deeper.

'Do you have any family out there, Jared?'

I had touched a raw nerve.

He paused, toying with the idea of telling me, and then said, 'No, Miss. I got no family.'

I sat quietly, inviting him to say more.

'I haven't got any brothers or sisters, none that I know of.'

He drew in another long breath.

'I grew up in care.'

His words lingered in our silence.

Since arriving at Huntercombe, I'd treated a number of boys who had been brought up in care homes, and some of their stories broke my heart. Their stories of physical abuse – and sometimes worse – emotional abuse, and trauma were harrowing.

How could poor Jared get to 18 and not have anyone on this earth who cared about him?

I thought about my two sons, and how lucky they were to have a mum and a dad who loved them.

I wondered if the reason why so many of the boys I saw in the prison were already young fathers themselves was because they longed for a family more than anything.

It got me thinking about how Jared might have acquired those atrocious scars on his back. From his childhood? Coming from a disadvantaged background didn't excuse Jared committing a crime, but I could understand how it might have taken away his self-worth enough that he didn't care what he did with his life. If nobody loved him, he probably struggled to love himself.

I wondered if there was something I could do to help him sleep. I couldn't prescribe him pills, but I chatted through some alternatives.

'Do you like reading?' I asked. A lot of the lads in

Huntercombe couldn't even read or write, but I was confident that Jared was quite literate from the way he expressed himself.

His eyes seemed to awaken at the mention of books. 'Yeah, I like to read. But sometimes I get my letters the wrong way around. It takes me a long time, and it drives me mad.'

'So not something that would be restful and send you to sleep, then,' I said, trying to think up other calming activities.

'I like to write though, Miss,' Jared confessed.

That wasn't something I heard of a lot in Huntercombe – and it seemed like a passion I could encourage to try to help improve his confidence.

He looked thoughtful. 'When I can't sleep I write down what I'm thinking.'

I thought back to that sleepless night after the argument at my old practice. Writing away until the dawn broke, changing my life with every word.

'Writing helps me get things off my chest,' I said. 'And I can feel much better when I put the pen down. So next time you're feeling overwhelmed, and want to cut yourself, why don't you try writing your feelings down first?'

Jared's voice trembled with emotion. 'Yes, Miss.'

I tried to catch his eye. 'Are you okay, Jared?'

'Yes, Miss.' He looked at me briefly before dropping his gaze back to the floor.

I told Jared that I had prescribed him painkillers for the next few days, and that he would need to collect them three times a day from the nurse. (Most prisoners were not allowed to keep drugs for self-administration, especially if they had a history of self-harm.) I suggested that he come and see me again if the backache continued.

As he walked out of my little consultation room, his shoulders were hunched; his feet dragged with exhaustion, from lack of sleep and misery. It was a heartbreaking sight, and for the first time I felt the presence of my patient lingering on in the surgery long after he had left.

*

My walks through the fields behind our house had always been cathartic, a way to process and unload my thoughts, letting them drift away into the countryside air.

I stepped over the stile in my Wellington boots, treading carefully so as not to skid on the wet slippery mud when I landed. I took a deep breath, filling my lungs with the crisp wintery air. I was walking through a paddock alongside two graceful horses that were tucking into a fresh pile of hay. They both looked up on hearing my squelching footsteps. One of them stared at me, intrigued, blowing hot, steamy air from its nostrils. It swished its tail a few times then returned to its munching.

How lucky am I to be walking freely through these fields? I thought. I'd trodden along that track dozens of times since I started working with the boys, but the contrast between their life, stripped of their freedom, and mine, had never been quite so obvious until then.

Those boys were teenagers – they should be going out and having fun, bringing friends home, having girlfriends, or boyfriends, being looked after. Instead they were banged up behind bars and it seemed so sad and wrong.

I felt unsettled by the thought of Jared, of what it must feel like to be locked away inside a tiny cell, knowing there was no one on the planet who cared about you. No one who would really miss you. No one to lean on when things got tough. He was one of many boys inside Huntercombe who had never known what it was like to have a family. He had left quite an impression on me.

Hearing Jared's story cast a shadow on the affluent world I'd known for so many years. The materialistic things I may once have thought were important suddenly seemed so trivial on hearing the 18-year-old's struggles. I realized more than ever that all that really mattered in life was feeling loved and secure.

A gust of wind hurled itself in my direction. I braced myself against its bite, hoping it would sweep away my mood so I could get a good night's sleep.

*

It seemed I had made as much of an impression on Jared as he had on me. One week later, he was back in my surgery, but with a slight confession.

'There's nothing really wrong with me, Miss,' he said.

I looked up in surprise, wondering why he had come to see me. 'Oh, well how can I help you then?'

He reached his hand inside his tracksuit pocket. I heard a rustle as he pulled out a scruffy piece of white paper.

I could see scribbles in all directions.

'I did what you said: I wrote down my thoughts. I made an excuse to see you so I could show you what I've done.'

Jared's cheeks flushed with his confession.

'Oh, that's wonderful,' I said. I was thrilled that he had taken my advice, and I felt touched that he felt compelled to show me what he'd done.

'I'd love to read it.'

Jared leant forward clutching the piece of paper with, if I wasn't mistaken, pride.

I suppose I was expecting to read a list of chaotic thoughts. The ramblings of a confused teenage boy wanting to offload his mind before bed.

But as I quietly read the lines, and between the lines, I was moved to tears: Jared had written the most beautiful poem about his childhood.

It was sad. It was moving. It was tragic.

It was also very well-written. Yes, it had a few spelling mistakes, and letters jumbled back to front, but Jared clearly had a talent, an ability to express himself.

'That's beautiful,' I said, sweeping my tears away with my forefinger.

Jared stared at me, I think in disbelief that something he had written could have had such an effect on me.

And then I broke my first prison rule: I gave him a hug!

I just felt so overwhelmed with the desire to show him

someone did care. He wasn't alone. I wanted to encourage him to continue with his writing. I knew it meant an awful lot to him that I'd taken the time to bother to read it, to know that I believed in him when perhaps no one had believed in him before.

I suspect it may have been the first hug he'd had in a long time.

'I'm glad you liked it, Miss. I'm going to write another poem and show it to you,' he said, filled with enthusiasm. His big eyes sparkled with excitement.

Jared clearly wanted to better himself, and I instinctively wanted to help. I couldn't wait until the next instalment.

I had the pleasure of reading two more of Jared's poems. They described why he had trouble sleeping. They told of the memories that came to haunt him in the night. But what was just as pleasing as seeing his efforts was hearing that the writing did help a little with his sleep.

I could see he struggled a bit with vocabulary, and the mother in me wanted to help him improve it, so one afternoon, after work, I swung past WHSmith. I knew exactly what I was looking for: a dictionary and thesaurus.

I showed it to David when I got home.

'I just want to give him something to help him with his writing. I can tell that he wants to learn, and I know it's only small, but small changes could go a long way. If Jared starts believing he's good at something, it might give him the confidence to make something of his life.'

Throughout our marriage David has always been the

calm, steady, rational one, whereas I'm much more hot-headed and emotional. We balance each other out that way.

'Just remember these boys are troubled,' he said. 'I don't want you to get too disappointed if you don't see the changes you hope for.'

I gave him a giant hug, putting my arms around his waist.

'What's that for?' he said, wrapping his arms around me.

I snuggled into him and smiled up at him. 'Just for listening to me and being wonderful. You don't need to worry. I won't be disappointed. Even if Jared only looks at the book once, it will have been worth it.'

*

I had a spring in my step as I walked towards the formidable prison walls the following morning. I knew Jared had a matter of weeks left before his move to the next prison. I was pleased to think that he would now have something with him to help take his mind off things, if he struggled to sleep in his new cell.

I hugged the large book into my chest as I waited for the thick metal door to slide back. My heart was skipping with excitement as I imagined Jared's face when it was handed to him.

'Morning, Doc,' said Joey, one of the prison officers, as he stuffed his bag into the locker.

A huge smile spread across my face. 'Just the man I wanted to see!'

'Uh-oh, what have I done?' Joey winked at me.

He was a big guy. His white shirt clung tightly to his belly, revealing tiny squares of his skin and hair where the fabric stretched apart at the buttons.

I asked him if he would be able to pass on a present from me to one of the boys on his wing, to Jared Keane.

'Keane?!' he exclaimed. 'The lad who's moving in a few weeks?'

I held out the book, still smiling.

Joey blinked a few times, lost for words.

'It's not the most exciting of presents, I know,' I giggled.

Joey continued to stare at it, then sighed deeply as he ran his hands backwards and forwards over his head.

'I don't know how to tell you this, Doc, but I can't give him the book. It's against the rules.'

I stared at Joey, crestfallen.

'But . . . why?'

Joey explained that giving Jared a present could be seen as conditioning, a term used to describe when inmates corrupt staff members and persuade them to smuggle things into the prison for them, including drugs and other banned items such as phones. My gift could be seen as a potential precursor to more serious contraband.

I snapped. 'Oh, for goodness' sake! It's just a book.'

'Rules are rules, Doc,' Joey shrugged. 'He'll have to wait until he's released to have it.'

'From the next prison?'

'Afraid so.'

I was so disappointed. I felt so deflated. The book would remain unopened amongst Jared's possessions for another three years. I wanted him to know that I believed in him, and cared about him.

I had to accept the rules of the prison, even though I found it very disheartening. I wanted to help him, but sometimes it was impossible to help people in prison.

The blocking of the book also highlighted another problem – trying to stop myself from getting too attached. Unlike in my old practice, where I would see the same faces, day in and day out, over the years, and could follow their progress to find out what happened to them, I had to wave goodbye to these teenagers with no idea of how the rest of their lives would pan out.

It mattered a lot to me to know whether I'd helped people. But being a prison doctor often meant that I'd never know.

I couldn't forget Jared. Every so often I thought of him, and of the choices he might have made, as I continued with my regular sessions in Huntercombe.

Did he continue with his poetry?

Did he find peace at night?

I carried on working there, and also became involved in a project working for the Primary Care Trust to try to improve end-of-life care.

One day it was announced that the prison was due to close. There were rumours that it might reopen as an adult Cat C prison, but nothing was confirmed, and so my time there came to an end.

However, I realised that I was in need of a bigger challenge. I wanted to entrench myself deeper within the prison system – to do the best I could within the limitations I had. I wanted to see if I could have more of an impact on the people I was dealing with. I suppose I was still searching for a purpose.

So, at the age of 55, when I could have been curling up on the sofa with a glass of wine and a nice book every evening, I applied to work as a doctor in one of the oldest and most notorious prisons in the UK.

PART TWO

The Scrubs
2009–2016

Chapter Seven

A stampede of prison officers crashed past my door. Their radios blasting 'Code Blue on A Wing'.

When Code Blue was called, everyone went: nurses, prison officers, doctors – a train of people racing along the landings.

Just in case I hadn't heard – though I could hardly miss the noise – nurse Sylvie banged on my door. 'Doc, Code Blue.' I grabbed my bag, shoved a pair of surgical gloves into my key pouch and joined the stream of staff flocking to A Wing.

A couple of weeks had passed and I was still finding my feet in the huge Victorian men's prison, Wormwood Scrubs, famously known as 'the Scrubs', with its five wings, A to E, each spread over four floors in West London. I was also adapting to the rude shock of coming from a relatively sedate institution, dealing with teenagers with minor medical ailments, to running between wings in a vast building that housed some very violent criminals.

I was overwhelmed with the size, the noise, the throbbing life of the place. A Code Blue was called for the most serious and often life-threatening emergencies, possibly a suicide.

I followed the stampede past the counselling rooms, as more radios crackled and more nurses and prison officers boarded our train.

'All out, all out, all stations. Code Blue on A Wing.'

I don't think any of us had a clue what we could expect to see at the other end.

Sylvie glanced back to check that I was keeping up.

I was familiar with the double gates that needed to be unlocked and locked to get from one area of the prison to the other. There were four gates that needed to be passed through in order to reach A Wing. Luckily, the person in front held the gates open for the next person to speed things up.

Clang! I heard the gates slam shut as I arrived onto the second floor of the massive four-storey wing

The stench of sweat lingered in the air from the prisoners who had been walking the landings minutes earlier. It was association time – the hour in the day when the prisoners are let out of their cells to mingle on the wing. But they'd been locked up prematurely to contain the Code Blue, and they weren't happy about it. Hundreds of fists pounding against the metal doors, exploding across the four floors.

I followed the human train along the landing, avoiding the stares of the prisoners leering out of the hatches in their green doors.

'Oi, let us out!'

'You're having a fucking laugh,' another man cried from across the wing.

I carried on marching to the beat of their fists, their eyes boring into me.

A deep voice, gravelly from cigarettes: 'I like the look of you, Doc.'

'Shut it!' barked the prison officer behind me, thumping the door for good measure. I was already ten strides ahead, focused on the crowd standing outside a cell. By the looks of sheer horror on their faces, whatever I was about to see must be truly shocking.

I pushed my way through them into what I can only describe as a bloodbath. There was blood everywhere – splattered across the walls, on the bed sheets. On the concrete floor, writhing in a pool of his own blood, was a young man with a massive slit across his throat.

Fortunately, a very competent young doctor called Mark was already there, trying to stop the haemorrhaging. He had been working in the doctors' room nearby when the alarm sounded. The ambulance was on its way.

Mark was on his knees, crouched over the man, blood spurting onto his white shirt as he pressed both hands over the gaping wound.

What had the prisoner used to cause such a wound? A smuggled knife or razor? In that moment it hardly mattered.

I pulled on my surgical gloves and crouched opposite Mark. We both had our hands wrapped across the prisoner's throat, desperately trying apply enough pressure to stop the bleeding but not so much that we strangled him, as we were also having to press on his wind pipe.

It didn't help that he kept twisting and turning, spluttering words in a language I couldn't quite catch.

'I think he's Spanish,' Mark said. 'Can't speak a word of English.'

The prisoner started squirming again, my hands slipping from his throat.

'Goddammit, can't we get anyone to hold him!' I shouted.

The cell was already too small with the three of us inside. Two prison officers in the doorway grabbed his legs in an attempt to pin him down.

The pool of blood was growing by the second, spreading across the floor, creeping under my shoes towards the walls. Despite the amount of it, he must have narrowly missed an artery, otherwise he would already have been dead.

He suddenly stopped fighting us. The colour of his face faded to white, his eyes rolled to the back of his head.

Mark yelled, 'Where's that ambulance?'

It seemed to take for ever for the paramedics to arrive. With someone's life literally in our hands every minute dragged impossibly on, with both of us wondering whether he was going to die in that hateful little room.

I kept pressing on the wound. It looked like raw meat. The blood bubbled up around my fingers, streaming into the man's long dark hair, matting it in clumps. He was about 25 years old. Trying to end his own life when he'd barely lived, it was tragic. I didn't even know his name. All I could do was keep talking to him, trying to reassure him.

'You're going to be fine, we're going to look after you,'

I said as I continued to plug the wound. I don't think he could understand what I was saying, I just hoped the tone of my voice would soothe him.

Suddenly, he jolted back to life and started thrashing around again. It was like trying to catch a slippery frog – there was so much blood everywhere.

'Will someone please hold him down?' Mark shouted. He knew it was no one's fault the cell was so small, but we were feeling the pressure, the enormous strain to keep this young man alive.

'Clear the decks, stretcher coming through!'

At last! Help had arrived, and relief washed over me. We had literally been fighting to hold on to a man's life. The weight of that, the pressure . . . The knowledge that we were about to pass that responsibility on, and to people with the space and facilities to manage the burden more easily, made me light-headed.

The people hovering outside parted to make way for the paramedics. There was so much blood on the floor now, the two men had to be careful not to slip.

The prisoner was completely still again as the paramedics prepared to move him on to the stretcher.

His head rolled to the side, his eyes were opening, closing, opening . . . and then staying closed for longer each time. He was fading. The paramedics counted down the lift on to the stretcher.

'One, two, three!' They heaved the prisoner sideways while I continued to press on the wound.

Just when I thought he had finally died, his eyelids opened. He looked directly into my eyes, staring at me with the most intense gaze. The only thing I could think was *Poor bugger, the last thing you're going to see is me!*

He clearly had other ideas, as he started struggling again like a caged wild animal. I wasn't sure if he was attempting to make a run for it, or if he was trying to stop us from saving him.

We pinned him down as the paramedics tightened the straps around his arms and legs. I wanted to scream. 'We've tried so hard to keep you alive, and you're killing yourself with every movement. Just lie still!'

But I had to remind myself: dying was, it would seem, exactly what he had wanted. I watched the paramedics carry him off along the landing, hoping for the best. They continued to apply pressure to the wound and get him to hospital as quick as possible. The wound was far too deep and extensive for a quick patch-up. He would almost certainly need a blood transfusion, that's if he even survived the journey to the hospital.

The banging from the prisoners was louder than ever, but a deathly silence had fallen across the crowd in and outside the cell. We all looked at each other, stunned.

Finally, Mark spoke, quietly thanking everyone for doing the best job we could have possibly done. We all shared the same sense of overwhelming relief that we had managed to keep the young man alive.

We then began to try to find out more about him . . . Who

was he? How long had he been in prison? What was his story? Was he on an ACCT book, or was his act of self-harm completely unexpected?

Nobody knew the answers. He had only been in the Scrubs for a few days. He hadn't needed to see a doctor, and as far as the staff knew, he was a foreign national on remand for burglary, waiting for sentencing.

The prisoner's cell mate, who had raised the alarm, was in just as much shock as everyone else.

He was a half-Asian guy, with a goatee beard and a shaved head. He must have been on remand, too, because he was wearing his own clothes rather than the grey prison tracksuit handed out to those who had been sentenced for their crime. Just over 60 per cent of the prisoners at the Scrubs were on remand – waiting to hear how much time they would have to spend behind bars. He had a thick cockney accent.

'I've been coming here for years and years. I've been in and out of prison since I was 17, but oh my days, I have never seen anything like that,' he said, staring in disbelief at the blood.

'Did he seem distressed or agitated?' I asked. I was still struggling to get my head around the idea that someone could suddenly just turn and slit their own throat.

His cell mate shrugged, kicking his foot against the wall. 'Nah, he was quiet, kept himself to himself, hadn't been causing me any problems. But then I wouldn't know because I couldn't understand what he was saying, anyways.' He coughed harshly. 'So who's going to clear this up then? 'Cos I ain't touching that blood.'

One of the prison guards stepped in. 'All right, all right, the Doc doesn't have time to hear about this,' he said and ushered him along the landing.

As everyone dispersed, I asked Sylvie if I could go to the loo. I was still being chaperoned everywhere until I had my own set of keys, which meant I needed someone to unlock the bathroom every time I needed to go.

We both walked in silence back towards the Healthcare block, still digesting what had happened. I didn't really need the loo, I just had this overwhelming urge to clean my hands. Even though I'd been wearing protective latex gloves, I could still envisage the blood on my fingers, hard to forget the feeling of its warmth and stickiness as it began to congeal.

I'd been in the ladies for a while when Sylvie called out.

'Are you all right in there, Doc?'

I'd slipped into a bit of a trance, letting the cold water wash over my hands, watching it swirl down the grimy plughole. My mind flashing back to the blood spurting out of the man's throat.

I was still a million miles away, trying to process what had happened, when Sylvie called out to me again.

'Doc?'

'Just coming,' I replied.

I looked up at my reflection in the mirror. My complexion was almost as ghostly white as the prisoner who slit his throat. My shirt was smeared with blood. On my face, splatters of blood! I rubbed furiously at the specks on my cheek with my forefinger.

Sylvie popped her nose around the door. 'Doc?'

I drew a long breath.

'Yes, sorry, just needed to clean myself up a bit. Ready to go now!'

Sylvie said that everyone involved in the suicide attempt had to head over to the governor's office for a debrief. 'It's standard procedure after a major incident,' she explained.

I was yet to properly meet the Number One Governor. The prison was so large it had a lot of governors, and they could be spotted easily amongst all the officers in uniform because they wore civvies.

I took one last look in the mirror, ran my hands through my cropped hair, took another deep breath and said, 'Yes, let's go!'

We walked across to the Admin block and a large meeting room where the governer was waiting. Soon we were all assembled, seated around the large conference table.

The governer thanked everyone for the part they had played in the incident, and asked if anyone had any concerns or comments about how things had been handled. He then said that if anyone felt traumatised by what they had seen they could go home early.

Nobody took him up on the offer. The day our response to seeing trauma was to walk away, well . . . that would be the last day we had in that place.

I normally would have listened to the radio on the drive

home, but I didn't want any noise cluttering my thoughts. Instead I let my body melt into the car seat, relaxing my limbs into the padded leather. All I could think about was getting back, slinging my clothes into the washing machine and jumping in the shower.

The sky turned grey and a little drizzle started to splash against my windscreen.

I wondered if the young man would survive. The last update I had heard from the nurses was that he had been taken to St Mary's Hospital in London, and was in a stable but critical condition. It was a miracle he was still alive.

I couldn't help thinking about Jonathan. How all those years ago I'd talked him out of slitting his throat. I'd been so shaken up at the horror of how I would have coped, if he had gone through with it. Now, so many years later, someone had actually done it and I had been there to help.

I had a terrible feeling it might not be the last time. I had chosen to step into an underworld where brutality was a way of life.

Maybe the young man hadn't meant to try to kill himself. Perhaps he just felt so desperate and overwhelmed with being in prison that he didn't know what else to do. I hoped and prayed that we had all saved him from making an irreversible, fatal decision.

Chapter Eight

I'd done it again. I'd woken up seconds before my 4.30 a.m. alarm started bleeping. But not soon enough to switch it off.

David groaned at the noise and rolled over.

I slipped from the bed and tiptoed to the bathroom. The birds outside were already awake, chirping, looking forward to the summer sunrise in an hour or so. I found it hard to be that enthusiastic so early in the morning. I needed a refreshing shower to jolt me into the day ahead.

I'd been getting up at the crack of dawn so I could miss the rush-hour traffic into London. I pulled into the Scrubs car park at 6.45 a.m. at about the same time that the officers and the nurses from the night shift were finishing. I was starting to recognise the same exhausted faces as they trudged towards their cars while I passed them on the way in.

There is probably no prison entrance in the UK more recognisable than Wormwood Scrubs, with its iconic brick and white stone towers and the huge wooden door.

It was built by convicts between 1874 and 1891, next to the 165-acre open space in Shepherds Bush, West London, known as Wormwood Scrubs. Back then, it was seen as massively progressive for its time. It was the first prison to use a 'telegraph pole' layout, whereby the wings were positioned in parallel blocks, arranged north to south so that every cell received sunlight, and designed to allow maximum circulation of fresh air, thereby minimising the spread of infection. The 'telegraph pole' plan provided a model for subsequent English prisons, such as Bristol and Norwich, and was closely copied by the second largest prison in France, Fresnes, and prisons across the USA. During the Second World War the jail was evacuated, and cells were used as secure government offices, including for MI5.

Today, the Scrubs is a Category B prison, housing 1,279 male prisoners over the age of 18 across its five wings. Occasionally the status is raised to Cat A, if an extremely dangerous prisoner is in residence while awaiting onward transfer. There are four categories of prison, ranging from Cat A, the highest security, to Cat D, or open prison, where the inmates can go out on day-release work, and sometimes have weekends at home.

Over the years it's held serial killers and celebrities behind its high brick walls. Some of the famous roll call includes Britain's most violent prisoner, Charles Bronson, who was moved to another jail after strangling the governor of the Scrubs. Moors murderer, Ian Brady, worked as a barber, cutting hair for inmates and staff in the 1970s. Rolling Stones guitarist Keith Richards was briefly locked up on drug charges. *EastEnders* star Leslie Grantham, better known as Dirty Den, served time in the Scrubs for killing a taxi driver in Germany in 1966. And just before I arrived, Babyshambles singer Pete Doherty had been at the Scrubs for fourteen weeks for breaching his probation.

I realised that during my time in the Scrubs I might meet a high-profile prisoner, but I didn't really think that I would find them any more or less interesting than the fascinating people I was already dealing with on a daily basis.

The history of the place oozed out of the walls. I could almost imagine the ghosts of prisoners past floating along the long corridors and up the dilapidated stairs, or lurking around the church outside B Wing.

I was past the gatehouse and inside the prison walls. The walk to B Wing looked like a rubbish tip – the pathway strewn with food, clothes, shoes, anything the prisoners could chuck through the small openings in their cell windows. I presumed they did it to make a nuisance of themselves, anything to annoy the prison officers, even though it was actually their fellow prisoners who had to clean up their mess. Red bands, they were called – the prisoners who were seen as more trusted and given enhanced status. They were awarded duties and access to areas other prisoners couldn't go, such as the expanse of open land between the wings and the prison gates.

I stepped over some foul-looking food, only to disturb a rat foraging on a stale baguette. He scuttled off half a metre and then started chomping on something else, his nose twitching with delight. He wasn't the least bit perturbed by my presence, just another annoying human getting in the way of his important rat business.

It wasn't a secret that the Scrubs was infested with rats and cockroaches, but it came as a bit of a shock when I first saw it for myself. An old building with ancient pipes and sewers, and rubbish strewn everywhere, it was hardly surprising it was a playground for vermin. I wondered how the prisoners felt, lying there at night with all that movement in the dark . . .

It was early but the temperature was already rising. The smell inside didn't bear thinking about – all that sweat and overcooked food.

But first, sleep. I had established a nice little routine whereby I was through security by 7 a.m., which left me time for a nap before I started work at nine. Essential, as I usually didn't finish until 10 p.m. I'd found the perfect spot for a snooze in one of the small rooms in the Seacole Centre, an area between the doctors' office and A Wing focused on mental health. It was completely deserted in there until the sessions started at about 9.30 a.m.

I reached up and pulled down my big black holdall, which I stored on top of one of the cupboards. It contained everything I needed for the perfect nap: a sleeping bag, and my neck rest, which I used for long-haul flights. I pushed three of the chairs together to form a make-shift bed. It was better not to look too closely at the blue-cushioned seat and back, and just roll my sleeping bag out before I could see the grimy stains. I was inside my cosy cocoon and asleep within minutes.

My alarm blared for the second time that morning. I wriggled myself out of my sleeping bag, yawned, stretched and slipped my feet back into my shoes, ready for the long day ahead.

The boy's prison felt like a holiday camp compared with the Scrubs. As duty doctor, my new role meant I could be called out to anywhere in the prison, at any time, for any medical crisis. It was fast-paced and varied.

At Huntercombe I'd never visited the cells, or the wings, as I just saw patients in the consulting room in the Healthcare department. At the Scrubs, I was going everywhere. It was much more challenging, far more exhausting, but very exhilarating.

Working in the Scrubs was a case of sink or swim. After a month in the job, my little naps were helping me swim, as were the lovely staff who had welcomed me into the prison. I was getting to know Sylvie a little more, as she was still escorting me around the prison while I waited for my key training from Security.

While grabbing a tea in the tiny communal kitchen, Sylvie shared some of the gossip.

'One of the nurses has just come back from a few months' compassionate leave,' she said, looking left to right to check that no one was overhearing us. 'She was taken hostage by one of the prisoners.'

I was lost for words. Where? When? How?

'I don't know all the details,' Sylvie continued. 'Only that he kept her hostage for a long time in one of the clinical rooms.

'Did he hurt her?' I asked.

'Nah, luckily.' Sylvie blew on her tea to cool it down. 'Well, not physically anyway, you can imagine how she took it mentally.'

'No wonder she had time off work,' I said. 'I'm surprised she came back!'

'That's the thing with this place, Doc,' said Sylvie with a sigh. 'It gets into your bones. It becomes just as much a home to the staff as it does the prisoners.'

I'd never felt that way about HMP Huntercombe, but in the short time I'd been working at the Scrubs, I was beginning to understand. The intensity of the work brought people together like a family.

'So what happened to the guy who took her hostage?'

She shrugged. 'Not sure, probably spent a fair bit of time in the Seg, and more than likely would have had time added to his sentence.'

The segregation unit, or Seg as it was better known, was where the prisoners were locked up for twenty-three hours a day. They were detained there for various reasons, sometimes for their own protection, but usually as a punishment.

'So you didn't fancy working at a women's prison, then?' asked Sylvie, changing the subject. 'Holloway didn't appeal?'

'It's horrible I have to think like this…' I paused, embarrassed.

'You thought a man would be less likely to beat you up than a woman?' Sylvie asked. I nodded, feeling somewhat ashamed.

'It's a fair point,' Sylvie said. 'Don't feel bad about it. We have to watch out for ourselves, don't we? If you want to know what Holloway used to be like, Governor Frake can tell you all about it.'

'Governor Frake?'

'She's head of Security, spent sixteen years at Holloway, when Myra Hindley was there, and Rosemary West. She's got a few stories to tell.'

٭

My first job of the day was to do the Seg rounds. I would then go to the First Night Centre to see any prisoners who had arrived the night before, and who had not yet seen a doctor. One of the main purposes of the clinic was to prescribe any medication that they may have been taking prior to custody. Some of the prisoners were inclined at times to exaggerate their symptoms in order to get certain medication, and it was my job to assess them without prejudice.

After finishing the clinic on the FNC I was asked to go and see someone on C Wing.

Sylvie was busy helping another doctor with his surgery, so one of the prison officers offered to chaperone me through the corridors and landings.

Terry had been working in the Scrubs for ten years. He seemed a gentle soul. His previous job couldn't have been more different: he used to develop photographs. A lot of the staff had lived very different past lives. One of the governors used to work for a big supermarket chain. Another had been a double-glazing salesman.

Terry had two children, both in primary school, and he could never wait to tell me about them. He was stocky, balding, with a goofy grin and shrewd blue eyes.

He unlocked the double gates into C Wing. 'After you, madam,' he said with a smile, locking the gates behind us.

The acrid smell of sweat was stronger than ever. It was Tuesday, laundry day. Piles of grubby socks, tracksuits and boxer shorts were piled high on the floor. I carefully stepped over them as I followed Terry.

There was a buzz of excitement in the air. The prisoners, milling around on their association hour, seemed a lot noisier than usual. The explosive sound of snooker balls smacking against each other echoed through the wing. I peered over the edge of the landing at the small group of guys who had gathered around the snooker table. They were egging each other on with heated expressions, and the air was filled with expletives.

Terry kicked a pile of clothes from his path with his big black boot.

'Everyone's a bit overexcited. It's Canteen Day.'

Canteen Day was a good day for the prisoners, as every week the food, drink and cigarettes they had ordered would be delivered by the canteen staff. All the orders were transported in large blue trollies, and the sight and sound of them rumbling along the landings soon became very familiar to me.

The list of choices included crisps, soft drinks, biscuits, chocolates, pot noodles and cigarettes. The canteen was a small independent business within the prison, and deliveries happened in the evening when all the prisoners were locked behind their doors.

'I've seen fights break out over a chocolate bar!' Terry laughed.

I could imagine they did. A piece of Cadbury's Dairy Milk must seem like the most precious thing in the world, when you have to wait a week to have it.

That and their phone calls to friends and family.

Prisoners were queuing up along the landing to use the communal phone, tensions rising as some feared that association hour would end before they'd taken their turn.

I could feel their angry eyes watching me as we squeezed past.

Terry looked over his shoulder. 'Can I give you a piece of advice, Doc?' he asked. I had a feeling he was going to tell me anyway.

'You've got to walk with confidence in here.'

I straightened my back.

'Some of them will want to take advantage of you,' Terry continued. 'So you've got to show them who's in charge.'

I pulled my shoulders back.

'Thanks for the tip,' I said. It was horrible to think I was being watched so closely. That people were looking for chinks in my armour.

We were suddenly brought to a standstill by an almighty cheer, followed by whistling and clapping and shouting.

One of the prisoners had thrown himself onto the netting strung between the landings. It was there to stop people jumping to their death, but this chap was bouncing around, up and down, as if he was on a trampoline, waving his arms in the air, soaking up the applause.

'Danny, Danny, Da-nny!'

The whole wing rushed to hang over the railings, chanting and cheering.

Danny was having a great time doing a bouncing lap of victory. It felt like we were at a football match, until a booming voice cut across the din. 'Get off, you idiot! Now!'

Standing on the opposite landing, with her hands on her hips, was a woman with cropped brown hair, wearing what looked like a men's black suit.

'That's Governor Frake,' said Terry. Head of Security for the prison, I remembered Sylvie telling me.

The chanting and clapping continued. But the governor had a surprisingly calm look on her face, as if she wasn't the least bit perturbed by the uprising and was very much in control of the situation.

'How to make yourself unpopular!' said Terry, nodding towards Danny.

'What do you mean?'

'Just watch.' Terry smirked, crossing his arms and leaning back against the wall, as if he was waiting for the real show to begin.

My ears nearly exploded with the sound of the alarm, and so did the prisoners' tempers.

'Oh fuck off!'

'You've got to be fucking kidding me!' came the cries of the inmates.

One of the guys queuing for the phone punched his fist against the wall.

Terry sprang into action.

'Back to your cells, lads, c'mon move it.'

The other prison officers manning the wing did the same, ushering the disgruntled inmates back to cramped cells.

'This plonker's just robbed them of their association time. If I were him I'd get off there, sharpish, or he's in for a beating tomorrow.'

But Danny hadn't seemed to realise the consequences of his actions quite yet. He carried on dancing long after the music had stopped, much to the amusement of Governor Frake.

'I've got all day, mate,' she hollered. Her hand hovering over the alarm bell, waiting for him to give up.

'When you're ready.'

The mood in C Wing had now shifted from jovial to hateful as the incessant screeching of the alarm drove the freshly locked-up prisoners towards the edge. They started thumping their cell doors in protest. Swearing and screaming at Danny to get off the net.

The smile soon left his face as he realised his supporters had swapped teams. He began to crawl back. Terry was ready, grabbing him by the scruff of the neck and pulling him back over the railings.

Danny was looking sheepish and slightly fearful as he waited for Governor Frake to make her way over.

'What do you want doing with him, Gov?' Terry asked his boss. 'Shall I take him to the Seg?'

She slowly walked up to him. Her hands in both trouser pockets. The fabric on her oversized jacket bunched up at her elbows.

She stood centimetres from his face and looked him dead in the eye.

His gaze dropped to the floor, nervously, as he waited for her verdict.

'Nah, let him face the music tomorrow,' she growled. She then turned and marched off in the opposite direction, switching the alarm bell off on her way.

Chapter Nine

I had barely placed my bag down in the doctor's office when I was immediately summoned to an emergency on D Wing.

All the prisoners were locked in their cells, but there was a crowd of officers gathered outside a ground-floor cell.

'It's not good, Doc,' one of the officers muttered as I walked past.

I took a deep breath and entered the cell.

Lying in the half dark, in a crumpled heap on the concrete floor, was a man in his seventies. His wrinkly, sinewy body was covered in blood and bruises. There looked to be a discrepancy in the length of his legs; I imagined he had a fractured femur. His internal injuries could – in fact probably would – be considerably worse, possibly life threatening.

'There's an ambulance on the way,' said one of the officers.

The old man coughed violently, blood spraying out of his mouth.

I touched his shoulder lightly.

'Please don't try to move,' I said.

His skin was turning purple with bruising. His wispy white hair was soaked in sweat and blood.

I asked the officer if he knew why the man had been attacked.

'They found out what he was in for, Doc,' he said, giving me a knowing look. 'He's a nonce.'

The old man was a paedophile, I had suspected as much.

Some crimes and acts of brutality are so beyond my comprehension that the only way I can cope is to block off all thoughts of them. All I could allow myself to see was an old man who had been brutally beaten up. He must have been terrified when they came at him, herded into a corner where the security cameras would be blind to them, surrounded by a group of men he couldn't possibly defend himself against. He must have thought he was about to die. Perhaps he had been right.

I sorted out some painkillers for him and waited for the ambulance to arrive.

'Stand back,' one of the officers yelled. The paramedics were finally there. 'You need to go, Doc,' he said to me. 'Some sort of panic on B Wing.'

I didn't even have time to oversee the old man being carried off. I slung my medical bag over my shoulder and marched out.

*

It was only early afternoon and I was already feeling exhausted. The morning had been hectic, with a lot of prisoners kicking off, causing drama and adrenaline levels to rise. I peeled off my surgical gloves and tossed them onto the growing pile of medical waste in the pedal bin. I'd just stitched up a man who had taken a razor to his legs. Cuts like screaming mouths from knee to ankle. It was so heartrending seeing someone self-harm, and I wished I could do more than just patch them up.

I let out a sigh and made my way back to the gates of the Healthcare wing. Time for a coffee and a snack – I had worked through lunch again.

As I walked along, I heard someone behind me. I turned round, and to my utter disbelief, shuffling my way was the last man I'd ever expected to see again.

With the huge gash across his neck held together by staples, there was no mistaking the Spanish man whose throat I'd held together with my hands.

It was association time and so most of the prisoners were milling around. Some were waiting their turn to play pool on the small table while they watched the others play.

He was trying to catch up with me but he was a bit short of breath. Perhaps he was still a bit anaemic, so I took his arm and gently steered him towards a chair where he could rest.

He looked up at me with his big dark eyes, longing to say something but lacking the breath.

I couldn't help but stare at the huge gash. It was a miracle he was alive. He'd wear the scar tissue like a scarf for the rest of his life.

I rubbed his arm. 'It's okay,' I smiled, trying to calm him.

He closed his eyes for a moment, just as he had done when I thought I was losing him, and then opened them wide, staring intensely into mine. Clutching his throat with his left hand, he mouthed, 'Thank you.'

My heart filled with joy. There's always a worry, when you save someone who has tried to kill themselves, that they'll hate you for it. I speak from sad experience.

I squeezed his hand and smiled – a universal expression that wouldn't be lost in translation. All the ups and downs and exhaustion of the day were suddenly worth it.

I held his words close as I walked away. They would be armour to throw on whenever feelings of self-doubt crept in.

'You need help with that, Doc?' Sylvie spotted me waiting for someone with a key. I nodded, overjoyed to see a friendly face.

I glanced at my watch. I had ten minutes before I needed to be at my security training meeting, where I was hopefully going to be handed my own set of keys. I was still new and yet these last few weeks had been the most traumatic, but also some of the most rewarding, of my life.

*

My ears were ringing with all the information that had been passed on to me over the previous two hours. All the new staff and agency workers, like me, had been cooped up in a room, learning about prison security. I'd discovered that a seemingly innocent piece of chewing gum could be used by the more ingenious prisoners as a means of escape – by taking impressions of an officer's keys. Under no circumstances was I allowed to bring it into the prison. Same went for Blu Tack – which explained why some cells smelt minty, as some of the prisoners used toothpaste as an alternative to stick their pictures on the walls.

Also on the banned list were spiral-bound notebooks. If the spiral fell into the wrong hands, a prisoner could use it to pick a lock.

Obviously, mobile phones were forbidden.

'They may look harmless enough,' the officer presenting the security talk said. 'But don't be fooled. Phones can be as lethal as the drugs that are smuggled in. They can be used to carry out criminal activity, to harass victims, to set up drug deals, and they can also be used as currency in the prison. An old Nokia mobile would go for £300 to £400!'

A little gasp of astonishment was let out by everyone.

After a fascinating talk, during which I learned all about contraband and all of the strict security rules I needed to obey, I was finally going to be allowed to draw keys.

I would be given a black circular piece of plastic with a number on it, called a tally, which I would hand in at the gatehouse in the mornings, in exchange for the exact combination of keys I would need to pass in and out of the clinical rooms and the wings. I wasn't allowed keys for the cells. If I needed to visit a prisoner in their room, for whatever reason, I would have to ask an officer to assist me.

But the really important message was left until last.

The officer took a deep breath before hammering home the point. 'Under no circumstances, and I mean *no* circumstances' – he raised his finger – 'are you to inform the prisoners who have been given hospital appointments, when their appointment is or where.'

A few of the nurses gave a knowing nod, while the rest of us were looking sideways at each other, a little perplexed.

He cleared his throat. 'As some of you know, last year what should have been a simple transfer to Hammersmith Hospital, ended in tragedy.'

Those whispering at the back of the room suddenly fell silent.

'A prisoner inside for armed robbery convinced one of the doctors that he was so poorly he needed to be referred to hospital to see a specialist. Unfortunately, he managed to find out the date, time and location of the appointment, and then tipped off his mates. Three of our officers were ambushed outside the hospital by men wearing balaclavas, pointing guns at their heads.'

The room was now deathly quiet as we all tuned in to the story.

The officer paused for a moment, rubbing his forefinger above his eyebrow, as if he was struggling a bit to come out with the next part of his story. We were hanging on to his every word.

'The men told our officers that they would shoot them, unless they released their friend. Obviously our boys took the cuffs off, because no one is worth dying for.'

Everyone murmured in agreement.

'We caught the guy after a couple of days on the run, and he got a few years added on to his twelve-year sentence. The police found one of the ambushers, but not the other.'

Someone from the back asked, 'What about the prison officers, were they unharmed?'

The officer telling the story paused for even longer this time, and I had a terrible feeling the answer wasn't going to be a 'happily ever after' ending, otherwise he wouldn't be telling it.

The officer reached for his glass of water behind him on the desk, which had stood untouched until then. He took a careful sip. 'Unfortunately the incident ended the careers of those involved, and we lost three excellent officers. Tragically, one of them became so depressed and anxious he even attempted suicide.'

A silence fell. I was just as lost for words as anyone else.

'So that, ladies and gents, is why we don't like to send anyone to hospital, unless it's a life-or-death situation – especially on a Saturday or Sunday when we are more likely to be short-staffed. And if they do have a hospital appointment, they must *never* be told of the date or location in advance.'

The warning was heavily directed at me and all the other healthcare workers in the room. It was unsettling to think that our decisions could come at such a high price.

'So please, make sure that you keep any information regarding hospital appointments under your hat, right up until the last minute. That way there will be no time to plan an ambush.'

And just as he was concluding his talk the alarm sounded.

Chairs screeched as everyone got up and dispersed. I went straight over to the gatehouse to get the tally, so that I could exchange it for the same numbered set of keys, but the keys I was given felt heavily loaded with responsibility. I couldn't even begin to imagine what it must have felt like for those officers to be held at gunpoint. To see their lives flashing before their eyes. Choosing whether to let a prisoner escape, or risk being killed, was a million miles away from the kind of decisions I used to make in my cosy GP practice.

It was going to take more than a horror story to put me off though. I attached the keys to the chain and tucked them in the leather pouch on my belt, and decided that the best way to get through life in a prison was not to think about it too much, not until I really had to.

Chapter Ten

It was a sorry sight, watching the new prisoners arrive at the Scrubs, dragging their large see-through plastic bags filled with all their possessions.

Sitting in the doctor's room in Reception, I could hear the bags sweeping along the corridor outside. They shuffled into the large holding cell opposite, the heavy sound of the door locking behind them. There, they'd wait to be screened by the nurses. The diversity of people coming from the Crown and magistrates' courts into prison varied enormously. It was like the A&E department of a hospital. I didn't know who was coming through those doors, nor what state they would be arriving in. I had to brace myself for everything. It could be rude, aggressive men, who were withdrawing from drugs and alcohol, many of whom were frequent attenders, or people who had never been in prison before, who could be nervous and shell-shocked. People from all ethnicities and walks of life, from wealthy, high-profile people to the homeless. Many of them shared the same shock and horror of being in prison – apart from some of the homeless men, who were happy to be in prison, just so that they would have food and shelter. The majority however, were very anxious. Occasionally some of them broke down and cried when they sat with me, knowing they were out of sight of the other men.

The new arrivals were screened by the nurses first, and there were usually two, sometimes three working the evening shift.

At 8 p.m. everyone had to move from Reception on the ground floor, to the First Night Centre on the fourth floor, to continue screening the new arrivals. So, along with everyone else that evening, I went up to the FNC until my shift finished at 10 p.m.

As usual, I had no idea what crimes the prisoners had committed, though the nurses would let me know, should the prisoner be accused of something particularly savage: murder, or a crime of extreme violence, as these prisoners would also need referring for a mental-health assessment.

I was warned about Azar by my dear friend Haj – one of the nurses – not because of the nature of his crime but because he was clearly in shock at being in custody.

I was reading through the Dubai man's notes when he was shown in.

I was a little taken aback by his presence. Despite being very unsure of his surroundings, the young man still carried himself with grace and elegance. He was tall, slim, with striking looks. I could immediately tell he came from money by the quality of his clothes. He was wearing a cashmere jumper and perfectly pressed chinos. His shoes looked of the finest quality leather.

His voice was soft and educated. 'Shall I sit here?' He pointed to the plastic chair adjacent to my desk.

His big brown eyes were wide, like a rabbit caught in headlights.

I smiled. 'Yes, come and sit down.'

I'd been warned that I should always leave my door open, and be the one sitting closest to it. That way I could escape quickly if I ever needed to. On the wall to my left was a big red alarm button in case of an emergency.

The room was small but clean. The thick, cloying smell of detergent hung in the air, a precursor to the cells the prisoners would be moved to next.

Azar looked around, nervously.

'I shouldn't be here,' he said trembling.

'Are you okay?'

He started shaking his head in disbelief.

'What am I doing here? I shouldn't be here!'

At that moment there was an almighty crash outside my room, followed by shouting and an ear-piercing scream.

'Get off me, get the fuck off me!'

Azar froze as he watched a man being dragged along the corridor by three burly officers, his legs kicking in all directions, his T-shirt yanked up around his neck, exposing his pale hairy body.

'Oh, Jesus!' Azar whispered.

I wished I could close my door to drown out the drama,

to keep him calm, but I knew that wouldn't have been a good idea.

Instead, I offered him the only thing I had to hand – my reassurance.

'You'll be okay, try not to panic,' I said.

Prisoners who were withdrawing from drugs, or who were on long-term medication for something like HIV, hypertension, or mental-health problems, would be given priority, as they would need to be seen before the end of the shift, so that their essential medication could be written up. I had the challenge of filling in the gaps until the prisoners' medical records were faxed through to the Scrubs, which usually took around twenty-four hours. That is, if they were registered with a surgery. Many of the homeless men were not.

From the notes that Haj had quickly made, I knew Azar was a diabetic on insulin. I didn't have much time, and I needed to get his medication sorted before he was shown to his cell.

'I'm going to be seeing a lot of you,' I smiled. 'The prison is very strict about not allowing inmates to administer their own injections.'

Azar looked even more horrified and panic-stricken, if that were possible.

'But don't worry, you will eventually have an in-possession risk assessment, and you will then be able to self-medicate and keep all your medication in your room. But initially the nurses have to administer it for you.'

'Okay,' he mouthed.

I went on to explain that all medication, except creams for any skin condition, and inhalers, had to be given out by the nurses on the wing until it was clear that a prisoner was going to take his medication regularly and reliably, and also that they were not at risk of overdose, nor of using the needles to attack another prisoner.

All colour had now drained from his face.

Azar suddenly stood up, only to wobble and fall back down into his chair.

'I know this must all seem very frightening, but you will be well looked after, I'll make sure your diabetes is under control,' I promised.

It must have been so shocking to be suddenly wrenched from his life of luxury and detained in custody. And then to be told that, on top of that, he no longer had control over his illness and medication. He must have been terrified; his world turned upside down.

I tried to keep him talking, to take his thoughts away from the brutal reality of the situation.

I looked him in the eye. 'Azar, you will be okay. Are you here on remand?'

He lifted his gaze.

'Twelve months on remand, but I might be extradited.' He quickly added, 'But I didn't do it.'

'It's okay, you don't need to tell me, I'm here to help you, not judge you. I don't have access to your prison records, just the medical ones, and that's the way I like it,' I explained.

'But I want you to know, they are accusing me of fraud but I'm innocent.'

That catchphrase 'everyone is innocent in jail' was now ringing in my ears.

'Any history of mental illness?' I continued.

'No.' He shook his head.

I softened my voice. 'Any history of self-harm? Do you feel like you might want to hurt yourself?'

He shook his head again. His perfectly styled black hair falling back into place each time.

Silence filled the room as I completed my entry on the computer. The medical records had recently been computerised, and I was still feeling my way around the system. Azar's eyes were transfixed on my hands, tapping away at the keyboard with my embarrassing one-finger-typing skills.

I was coming to the end of my shift, but despite feeling tired I wanted to find out more about Azar. He was clearly struggling so much to come to terms with being in prison.

'Do you have any family who you can turn to?' I asked.

He sighed deeply.

'I have a beautiful girlfriend. I have a loving family. I have a mother . . .' His voice faltered, trembling. 'I have a mother who is very disappointed in me. She thinks I'm guilty. She says she can't understand why I would have committed fraud, when we have so much money already.'

He was on the edge of tears as he looked up at the small barred window, and stared out of it, no doubt imagining the freedom on the other side.

He then turned to me. 'I'm from a very wealthy family, you see. We have companies and properties all over the world.'

Which was just as I had predicted. I suspected his crime must have been fairly serious, bad enough to warrant being refused bail – he would have had enough money to have paid for it otherwise.

'Well, hopefully they will come and visit you soon,' I said.

Azar nodded.

'I'm not sure if I can face my mother. When she makes up her mind about something, it's very difficult to persuade her otherwise.'

I nodded.

'I can't bear the thought of being without Jazmin.' His voice cracked again.

'Your girlfriend?'

'She's so beautiful!' he exclaimed, reaching into his bag for what I assumed was her picture.

Just as he was pulling out a little bundle of photographs, the officer in charge poked his head into my room.

'We got an emergency, Doc, someone you got to see.'

I looked at Azar apologetically as the officer ordered him out of the seat.

'Move it!' he said, gruffly. He was one of the three burly officers who had restrained the noisy guy earlier.

Azar looked panicky.

'It's going to be okay. Deep breaths if you feel over-whelmed,' I said as he was being led away. He looked back at me.

'Keep calm,' I mouthed.

And with that he disappeared. But I knew that, because of his diabetes and the length of time he was on remand, I would most likely be seeing a lot more of him, which pleased me as I'd warmed to him.

Chapter Eleven

One of the prison officers, Ed, needed my help.

He'd phoned the doctor's office asking me to come to the Seg immediately.

As I arrived, he was pacing around, looking anxious and angry. From the way he was behaving it clearly wasn't a Code Red or a Code Blue crisis, but nevertheless something serious had happened.

'Thanks for coming so quick, Doc,' he said.

I peered up the metal stairwell to the cells above.

'Where do I need to go?' I placed my foot on the first step.

Ed stopped me in my tracks.

'Not up there, Doc, we need you in the obs room.'

The observation room was reserved for prisoners who needed to be watched twenty-four hours a day on CCTV. There was nothing in the room at all.

Ed grimaced. 'Prepare yourself.'

I followed behind him, dreading what I might be about to see.

The door to the cell was open and I could see the backs of several officers crammed inside.

'So,' said Ed. 'This idiot has gone and stuffed some razor blades up his arse!'

I wasn't sure I'd heard correctly. 'Sorry, what?'

Ed explained that it wasn't as unusual as I might have thought. The prisoner was using the razors as a last-ditch attempt to prevent being transferred to another prison.

'By stuffing razors up his arse, he's effectively concealing a weapon, which he could then attack staff or inmates with. The other prison will refuse to take him if he's armed.'

I was speechless. The lengths that some of the prisoners went to was incredible. Prisoners might resist a transfer for a variety of reasons, such as not wanting to be moved far from their family, making it more difficult for them to visit. They may have enemies in the other prison, or possibly owe money to people there that they cannot repay. Some, on the other hand, may be dealing drugs and be owed money in the Scrubs.

This case must have been something along those lines, for the prisoner to have taken such extreme measures.

'Has he wrapped them in anything? Clingfilm?'

I hoped so, otherwise he could be bleeding internally.

'He won't say'.

I asked Ed if he had any spare surgical gloves. I'd used my last pair on a prisoner in E Wing, and hadn't had a chance to grab more. He disappeared inside his office then re-emerged with a large pair of black plastic gloves that looked a bit like gardening gloves. They would have to do. I'd tried to find some in the tiny Seg doctor's office, but there weren't any. I did, however, find a roll of disposable white plastic aprons. I pulled one off, tied it around my waist, and put on the gloves Ed had found.

In the observation room, the prisoner was kicking off again. The three officers inside were wearing restraint uniform – which looked like riot gear; thick black overalls and a black helmet with a visor to protect their faces.

A deep voice shouted, 'I'm staying here! I'm not fucking moving to that hell-hole! Try and make me and I'll fucking sock you one.'

Ed was having none of it. It was easy to tell why he was in charge of the Seg; no one messed with him.

'Shut it!' he shouted.

There was a foul smell in the small room. Their shouts bounced off the walls, becoming deafening.

'Don't kick me!' the prisoner shouted.

Ed sighed. 'No one's going to kick you, Clarke. The Doc's here; she's come to take the razor blades out of yer arse. Don't want you bleeding to death, do we?'

The prison officers parted, revealing a scrawny little man, writhing around on the floor like a worm. He was white, around 35 years of age, with tattoo sleeves on both arms.

He glanced up at me, standing in the doorway wearing an apron and two oversized black gloves. He suddenly froze with sheer horror. 'No!' he screamed. 'I'll take them out myself!'

Thank God for that, I thought (not that I'd have been permitted to do a rectal examination without his consent).

'Wise choice, mate!' said Ed.

I flashed Ed a relieved look as I pulled the gloves off, the latex making a snapping noise as it left my skin.

'Don't tell me you've got somewhere you'd rather be,' he joked as I headed for the exit.

*

As it was lunch time, I returned to the doctors' office. Zaid, one of the other locum doctors, was there, looking as stressed as I felt.

'I need a cigarette!' he said. 'Fancy keeping me company?'

'Definitely!'

We took it in turns to unlock our path to the courtyard outside Reception.

It was wonderful to be greeted by sunshine. I closed my eyes, craned my neck to the sky and bathed in the summer warmth, lapping up the fresh breeze.

'Not here, AB.' Zaid interrupted my moment of escapism. His nickname for me was my initials.

He took a left, leading me alongside A Wing. The narrow strip of land between the prison and its formidable walls reminded me of a wasteland in an apocalyptic film. Strewn with rubbish it was hardly a scenic view, but it was the best the Scrubs could offer.

Zaid reached into his pocket and pulled out a packet of cigarettes. He tugged one out of the box with his mouth, and cupped his hand around the end as he lit it.

We stood there in silence as he sucked the smoke deep into his lungs, his face a picture of contentment.

Finally, he spoke. 'So how bad has your day been so far?'

I rolled my eyes. 'I had to go to the Seg to see someone who had shoved razor blades up his arse.'

Zaid didn't seem the least surprised. He glanced at me sidewise, blowing a ribbon of smoke into the air.

'One of those,' he said, also rolling his eyes.

'How about you?' I asked.

'I had to attend a resuscitation on D Wing,' Zaid replied. 'Guy tried to hang himself. Didn't succeed. And then I had to see someone who self-harmed by swallowing a couple of batteries.'

We were both silent again for a moment.

It was a world away from the lunch-break conversations I'd had back at my old practice. I'd probably have been discussing the latest HRT medication, or new NICE guidelines.

Zaid broke into a smile, showing off his perfectly white teeth. 'While we're out here, come and look at this,' he said, beckoning me further into the wasteland.

'It's my favourite pastime,' he said as we stepped over the piles of rubbish.

There was a huge mound of earth, half a dozen rats whizzing in and out of it. They didn't even blink at our presence.

'Wow!' I said.

Zaid took a drag on his cigarette. We were both mesmerised by the sight of them scuttling to and fro. Most people would go somewhere nice on their lunch break. There we were, staring at vermin.

'Better get back to it.'

Zaid threw his stub onto the ground, crushing it out under his shoe.

'Seen this?' he said as we made our way back to the entrance gates. He pointed to a sign on the wall which I hadn't noticed before. In big red letters it said: DON'T APPROACH OR FEED THE FERAL CATS.

'Yeah,' he said. 'They've brought in wild cats to try and catch the rats, but they don't seem to be too good at it!'

When he'd gone I stood for a few more minutes in the sunshine. Then unlocked the gates and went back to work.

Chapter Twelve

One Sunday afternoon I was asked to see a young man on B Wing.

He had been ill for the past few days with diarrhoea and vomiting, and looked extremely unwell. He was clearly in a lot of pain as he struggled to get onto the examination couch.

He was a tall, slim Sri Lankan man in his early twenties.

I introduced myself, took a history, and then after looking in his mouth I gently placed my hand on his abdomen and found that it was rigid and very tender. He was feverish, pale and sweaty, and I suspected he may have peritonitis, possibly resulting from a ruptured appendix.

He needed to go to hospital as soon as possible, and so the nurse arranged an ambulance.

As I was typing a referral letter the deputy governor entered the room.

He was very intimidating. Always immaculately dressed in a smart suit, white shirt and plain tie, and he wore the shiniest shoes I have ever seen.

I saw the shoes before the face, and I knew it was him!

He was strict, well-spoken and an absolute stickler for the rules. In fact, I was so intimated by him that I usually looked at the floor whenever he was heading my way. Because his shoes were so highly polished that I could virtually see my reflection in them, I had nicknamed him Shiny Shoes.

He scowled, looked at his watch and then back at me.

'Doctor Brown,' he began, in his well-spoken voice. He always addressed me formally. 'The prisoner has been unwell for the past two or three days. Why are you sending him out on a Sunday afternoon?'

I understood the problems he was facing. He was already understaffed, and two officers would be needed to accompany the young man to hospital. He murmured something about having to shut three of the wings down if the prisoner went to hospital, which meant hundreds of men being deprived of their precious association time.

More pressure.

More guilt.

But this time I stood my ground, looked him firmly in the eye, and explained that the prisoner might have peritonitis, and could not wait until tomorrow to go to hospital, as it was potentially life-threatening.

The prisoner groaned, but lay very still, grimacing in pain.

Shiny Shoes put his hand in his pocket and narrowed his eyes. 'Doctor Brown, couldn't he simply have gastroenteritis? Aren't diarrhoea and vomiting symptoms of that too?' His tone was firm and icy.

A flame of anger flashed through me, and I repeated in

an equally icy tone that the patient needed to go to hospital today!

In that moment I hated my job. I was well aware of the risk of prisoners faking an illness so that they could try to escape, but I was sure that wasn't the case.

Silence. Eventually, Shiny Shoes glanced at the prisoner and then back at me. 'You're putting me in an awkward position here, Doctor Brown. You wouldn't be the first doctor to make a misdiagnosis.'

I remained silent but kept looking him firmly in the eye. It was a terrible position to put me in, but I wasn't going to be intimidated.

He radioed the switchboard, and confirmed that the young man would be going to hospital, and that the ambulance should be called.

'If you'll excuse me, Doctor Brown,' he said curtly, and then made a sharp exit.

As soon as he had left, I felt the pressure ease. I didn't dislike Shiny Shoes, and I knew he was also under an enormous pressure, and that he was very good at his job. I just wished he thought I was good at mine!

I went back to the man's side. He was retching and groaning, and the blue roll of tissue beneath him had almost disintegrated with sweat. I tried to reassure him that everything was going to be fine, but there was nothing I could do while we waited for the ambulance to arrive.

Soon two prison officers arrived at my door, one holding a pair of handcuffs.

'He doesn't look good, Doc!' the officer exclaimed, quickly handing the cuffs over to his colleague. 'You can be cuffed to him!'

'Don't worry, he's not contagious,' I told them.

They didn't look convinced.

'You're going to have to take my word for it,' I snapped. I'd had quite enough for one day of trying to convince people I was telling the truth.

*

It wasn't just the emergency hospital transfers that caused problems for the doctors. Getting prisoners to their scheduled hospital appointments could also be extremely difficult. Sometimes there simply weren't enough prison officers available to escort them. As a result, they would often miss their appointment, and have to have it rebooked, sometimes more than once, causing a further wait of maybe three to six months before they were seen. It made managing their illnesses much more difficult.

One day, on finding a prisoner I was concerned about had missed their appointment for the second time, I couldn't help but moan to Sylvie.

'It's not the Scrubs' fault,' I said. 'It's the lack of staff.'

She nodded. 'I've seen a lot of doctors leave because they get so frustrated by it. Coffee?'

I could have murdered one.

'Sorry, I can't,' I replied. 'I've got to go to the Seg and see someone who tried to set fire to his cell.'

Sylvie wished me luck and smiled encouragingly. 'Doc, don't let this place get to you.'

'I know. It just feels like an uphill struggle at times.'

*

To be locked in a very small cell for twenty-three hours a day must have been hard to cope with. Sometimes, when the prisoners were walking round the exercise yard outside the Seg, which was at a slightly lower level, I would see their heads bob up at the doctors' office window.

''Ello, Doc,' they'd shout, anything to start up a conversation, desperate for a bit of interaction.

Living in such extreme isolation obviously took its toll on some of the inmates, and occasionally caused them to suffer from anxiety and panic attacks. Others would compulsively pace around their cell, or clean it repeatedly, while others spent hours doing press-ups.

The prisoners in the Seg were seen on a daily basis by the duty doctor, accompanied by a nurse and a prison officer. They were also visited regularly by Chaplaincy and the Independent Monitoring Board. Whether they chose to see me when I came knocking was another matter.

The prison officer would lead the way, thump his fist on the hatch in the door to announce our arrival, open it to check all was okay inside, then unlock the door. Sometimes a shout came back, 'I'm, having a crap!' so we would move on to the next cell and return at the end of the round.

'Doc's here'.

I was not allowed to go in the room without the officer's permission. Most of the time I didn't need to.

Sometimes a prisoner wanted to engage, possibly to ask for medication. Often I was ignored completely. Occasionally, I might wish I had been, as a tirade of abuse was hurled at me.

If a prisoner was extremely dangerous, the door could not be unlocked and the consultation, if there was one, had to be conducted through the hatch. Even that was not always possible, if there was a risk of having urine or faeces thrown, or of being spat at. In that case the conversation would be conducted through the tiny gap at the side of the cell door. On the very rare occasion that a very violent man needed to be seen, a sign saying 'three man unlock' would be placed below the name and number outside the cell, and the door could only be opened when there were three officers outside the cell on standby.

Most of the prisoners would be lying on their backs, arms folded behind their heads as they stared at the ceiling, without saying a word. Others would hide under their sheets, and I would look to see if they were still breathing.

I was advised to not enter the dingy cells if I could help it. Ed told me it was better to stand at the door, protected by an officer. The lighting was very poor in the doorway, though, so if I needed to examine a prisoner for any reason, I would have to go towards the far end of the cell, where light came through the small window, but that was only if the officer allowed it.

I knew I was in for some trouble as soon as I walked onto the Seg that day. The banging of fists on the cell doors echoed up and down the corridors and over the two floors.

Terry was on duty. 'You've got your work cut out for you today, Doc.'

He chaperoned the nurse and me along the landing, the sounds of our shoes on the metal gantry drowned out by the noise of the prisoners' protest. I stood back as Terry knocked twice and then yanked back the hatch. He did not unlock the door; it was too dangerous.

'The Doc's here,' he shouted.

I gingerly stepped forward, bracing myself for what I was going to see in the cell. One of the challenging things about working in prisons was never knowing what might be waiting on the other side of the door.

In this instance, it was a young, skinny man, running up and down his cell, totally naked. He seemed to be completely wild, thrashing his arms around and shouting nonsense. He suddenly stopped in his tracks and locked eyes on me. He looked as if he was possessed. His eyes were fierce as he stared at me through the small hatch in the door.

'Nah, she can fuck off!' he barked, momentarily aware of our presence, before he continued his rant.

There was clearly no point trying to have a conversation with him.

I suspected he may have been using spice, a synthetic

cannabinoid that can have devastating effects on the user, before being moved to the Seg, which would explain his wild behaviour. He carried on running up and down his tiny cell, thumping his fists against the wall as he went, screaming a continuous stream of expletives.

Terry slammed the hatch shut as I walked on to the next cell. My heart went out to the officers working the Seg that day, as they certainly had their hands full. If he had used drugs, there was no way of knowing when he might calm down.

There was a particularly vicious batch of spice going around the prison at that time, and the effect it was having on people was terrifying. Some became acutely psychotic, others had fits, some lost consciousness.

Stopping drugs from entering the prison was a never-ending problem for the officers, especially Govenor Frake, who was in charge of Security.

Sometimes drug packages were chucked over the prison walls into the grounds, but most of those would be discovered by the prison staff – although some would be picked up by prisoners, sometimes even the red bands. A red band prisoner once confessed to me that he was being threatened by another prisoner, and told that if he failed to get the parcel one of his family would get hurt.

I also learned that drugs and phones were smuggled in on visits, and that Govenor Frake had once caught someone with three phones and a number of bags of cocaine in her vagina. 'It must have been bigger than a clown's pocket,' she'd said with a harsh laugh.

Another way spice was getting in was on letters addressed to prisoners, as it could be sprayed onto the writing paper, which was then cut into small pieces and smoked. I'd looked at Terry in disbelief when he'd first told me that, and I remember feeling quite naïve at the time.

Terry banged on the next cell door. 'Doc's here!' he shouted.

No reply.

'This one is a self-harmer. You'll be lucky to get anything out of him,' he informed me.

I peered through the hatch into the dark cell.

The man was sitting on his bed with his back against the wall, half in the gloom, half in the shaft of light coming through the window. He was Afro-Caribbean, his long black hair hanging loose past his shoulders.

His arms were glistening with what looked like blood.

I turned to Terry, perturbed. 'Is that blood all over his arms?'

Terry nodded. 'More than likely, Doc. You can't stop him. We've tried everything. It's like a bloodbath in there.'

'We need to open the door!'

Terry frowned. 'I don't mind opening it, but you'll have to wait at the door. He's in here because he's too dangerous to be anywhere else.'

Strangely, I wasn't afraid. I just wanted to check if he was okay.

Terry unlocked the door and the key scratched as it turned in the lock. He yanked on the handle, releasing the door. A sharp, sour smell of old blood blended with sweat poured my way.

The prisoner didn't even look up. Instead, he continued to slice at his already open wrist wounds with his overgrown fingernails.

Terry wasn't exaggerating, the cell was covered in blood. The sheets, the washbasin, he'd even smeared the walls with it.

'Can't you do anything to stop him?' I asked Terry.

He shrugged. 'It's impossible to stop him doing it. As soon as his wounds get stitched up he's at it again.'

I knew serial self-harmers would use just about anything to cut themselves – from their fingernails, to the edges of a yoghurt pot, to the metal of their bed frame. I also knew that they often reopened the same wounds over and over again to prevent them from healing. The question of why he was doing it was the biggest problem of all. I hoped Terry could give me some insight.

'He's Jamaican, waiting to be deported. He doesn't know when, could be months away, could be years.'

That's all Terry needed to say. I'd learnt that foreign national prisoners were some of the most volatile of all in the Scrubs. A lot of the prisoners I'd met were pretty pragmatic about their sentence – 'they've done the crime, they'll do the time' – but foreign nationals often didn't know what the 'time' would be, nor if and when they might be deported, and that made it very hard for them to cope. There was a high rate of self-harm amongst them, and some were full of hatred, bitterness and anger.

I glanced at the name underneath the prison number pinned to the door.

'Josef,' I said softly.

Nothing.

I wanted to try to get Josef to engage with me, and I hoped that even a brief conversation might help him to take the focus away from cutting his arms and his legs, and on to something else.

I said his name again, more gently. But still nothing. Instead he continued to pick at his cuts.

Terry stepped in. 'Doc wants to know if you need anything.'

Josef slowly turned his head towards us, staring blankly through his greasy strands of hair. His flat, empty expression was so sad and I really wanted to understand him and be able to engage with him. But Terry grew impatient, slammed the door shut and locked it.

He looked at me sympathetically. 'Warned you, Doc. He's a waste of time. Some people just don't want to be helped. He won't talk to anyone.'

I refused to believe that anyone was beyond help. I was determined to persevere, and to try my very best to show him that I cared and wanted to help him.

We arrived at the next cell.

'Mind the hatch, this one likes to throw shit!' said Terry.

I tensed, preparing to jump out the way.

Chapter Thirteen

'Doctor Brown, would you have a moment?' It was more of a command than a question. There was only one person in Wormwood Scrubs who addressed me in that way.

I slipped the keys I was about to use on the Healthcare gates back into my pouch, took a deep breath, and turned around to look directly at the deputy governor.

He cleared his throat. 'I just wanted to say, I'm sorry.'

It was hard to disguise my surprise.

'You were right to insist that the young man was taken to hospital. It was indeed a case of peritonitis.'

I'd already heard a report from the hospital stating as much, and that the prisoner had been so unwell he had remained in hospital for two weeks. I hadn't expected an apology from the governor himself though.

'Thank you.' I smiled. 'I appreciate you telling me that.'

The silence settled between us again, both of us unsure what to say next. I was rescued by Sylvie, who was dashing past.

'You're needed in B Wing,' she said, breathlessly.

I turned back to Shiny Shoes. 'If you'll excuse me.'

'Doctor Brown.'

He nodded in polite, old-fashioned recognition, and I chased after Sylvie into the adjacent wing.

'What's happening?' I asked.

'It's the prisoner with diabetes, that's all I know.'

*

Azar's diabetes had been difficult to control as the food in the Scrubs was often high in carbohydrates. Although the prison tried to provide a suitable diet for diabetic patients, it wasn't always available, and on many occasions his glucose level was so high the reading was 'Unrecordable' on the glucometer. This indicated that he was at risk of hyperglycaemic coma. Sometimes, too, due to the erratic diet and timing of his insulin, his sugar levels dropped too low, which could also lead to a hypoglycaemic coma.

But I'd never had to visit him in his cell before. It had to be serious if he was too unwell to make it to the nurses' room. One of the prison officers was waiting outside, ready to unlock the door for me.

'How bad is he?' I asked. I'd become quite attached to Azar.

'See for yourself, Doc.' The officer turned the key and opened the door.

Azar was perched on the edge of his bed, his body tense, his face dripping in sweat, his breathing fast and shallow.

A look of relief seemed to wash over him as he saw me enter his cell.

His big brown eyes were staring up at me, pleading for help.

Somehow, though, I did not feel this was diabetes related. I pulled out my stethoscope and listened to his heart and chest, while Sylvie checked his glucose level, which was normal.

His heart was pounding at speed, but at least the rhythm was regular. Coupled with his sweating, hyperventilating and the way he was behaving, it was more likely that he was having a panic attack.

I sat next to him on his bed.

'Don't be afraid,' I said. 'It will pass, and you'll feel back to normal again soon.' I was trying to reassure him; people can fear they're going to die during a panic attack.

I tried to get him to slow his breathing down by taking long, deep inhalations through his nose, and out through his mouth. I told him to copy me, breathing with him until, slowly, his breathing settled back to a normal rate.

As he calmed down, I looked around his cell. It was immaculate. The pictures of his family were hung in per-fectly straight lines. His clothes were folded so neatly they could have been on display in a shop. His toothbrush and toothpaste, razor and shaving foam were laid out within equal distance of each other. He was clearly obsessive about keeping things neat and tidy.

It struck me that Azar might suffer from obsessive com-pulsive disorder.

OCD is quite a common disorder, and can have

devastating and crippling effects on people's lives. Those who suffer from it often have an overwhelming urge to check things over and over again, perform certain routines or rituals repeatedly, and have obsessive thoughts. Commonly, someone suffering from OCD might wash their hands over and over again, or keep going back into the house to check all the electrics have been turned off before going out, or that the door is locked. Another typical symptom would be an obsession with cleaning, or having things lined up perfectly.

Often the OCD worsens when people feel anxious or stressed. When someone's life is spinning out of control, performing rituals or routines can be their way of scrabbling back some of that control. It wasn't hard to see why a prisoner might suffer from it.

'How are you feeling now?' I asked.

He nodded instead of speaking, his breathing now steady and his heart rate returned to normal.

'Don't worry. I'm not going anywhere. Just take your time,' I reassured him.

Azar screwed up his eyes tightly, trying to forget the world he was trapped in. I suppose a lot of the inmates close their eyes, wishing to wake up on the other side of the prison walls, often waking up in blind panic in the middle of the night when they realise where they are.

I waited patiently until he was ready to tell me what had made him feel so panicky.

A bead of sweat dripped into his eyes and he blinked it

away. He reached for the folded towel by his sink, dabbing his face dry.

He finally spoke. 'It's filthy in here!'

I didn't think that then was a good moment to break the news that his cell might have been the cleanest in the whole of Wormwood Scrubs.

'I'm always cleaning, but it's never clean enough.' He was on the edge of tears.

My heart went out to him. He'd been plucked from his lavish lifestyle and detained in custody. It must have been a dreadful culture shock for him, probably much more so than for a lot of the other inmates.

He couldn't control his fate – he was waiting to hear if he would be extradited. He couldn't control his diabetes. It seemed as if he was channelling all his frustrations into cleaning his cell, and it was getting the better of him.

He suddenly lurched forwards, grabbed a giant lump of soaked loo roll in his right hand, and began scrubbing a patch on the wall, so furiously the tissue quickly disintegrated between his fingers.

His breathing started to speed up again and it looked as if he was heading for another panic attack.

I touched his shoulder. 'Come and sit back down,' I said, being careful to keep my voice light.

'Do you have any wet wipes?' he asked, breathlessly.

I always carried a packet, because I too was pretty fastidious when it came to cleanliness. But it would have been frowned upon for me to hand them over to a prisoner.

Azar's eyes were pleading, and it seemed like such a small thing to do to help someone cope. I rummaged through my bag and passed Azar the last few wipes I had left.

As soon as he held them between his fingers he seemed to relax.

'Thank you! Thank you!' he was shaking, overcome with gratitude.

In truth, I could empathise. I was also inclined towards obsessively washing my hands, in part due to my job. I hated the thought of handling dirty keys all day long. One of the first things I did on arriving in the morning was to boil the kettle, put the keys in the sink and pour boiling water all over them.

Azar placed the wet wipes carefully on the side of his basin, no doubt ready to start scrubbing after I left.

It was such a small gesture on my part, but perhaps they would be of some comfort. I was not able to do much to improve the prisoners' lives, but sometimes little things seemed to make quite a difference. Many times I was told that just knowing that someone cared helped them to cope.

I stayed with Azar a little longer to make sure his panic didn't resurface, keeping our conversation light to avoid anything that might act as a trigger.

But he insisted on telling me that his lawyer was coming to see him in the morning to discuss his case. Although I'd seen him many times now, I still didn't fully understand what he'd been accused of. His case was very complex, and, quite frankly, I didn't particularly want to know too much about it.

His frown lifted as he said, 'And my girlfriend is coming to visit me the day after.'

'That's wonderful,' I said, beaming. I much preferred chatting about the positive things that carried the prisoners through their daily grind. A visit from a loved one, a hand-drawn painting from a child they could hang by their bed, a letter from a best friend or a partner. Those were the things that mattered in a place like the Scrubs.

I checked my watch. I was running late as I needed to see someone on A Wing before lunch, so I said my goodbyes, promising that I would refer him to the Mental Health Team to help him manage his OCD, and that I would see him again soon. I wished I had more time to spend with patients, but I always seemed to be in a rush.

'Try and stay calm,' I said. 'And if you find yourself feeling panicky again, do the breathing exercises.'

The help I could give him was limited, but I hoped that knowing I cared and understood a little of what he was going through was of some comfort.

*

I quickened my pace as I headed off to A Wing, hoping I wouldn't be called anywhere else before I got there, but running towards me were three nurses.

'Code Red, D Wing!' one of them cried.

I turned around and joined them.

It was the familiar panic. The adrenaline rush. The

apprehension of what was to come. Racing along the corridors, unlocking and locking the many barred gates, dreading what grim sight awaited us.

The nurse in front cleared a path through the prisoners who were wandering around during their association time. I could recognise many of the faces by now, and some I knew by name. They all knew mine, of course, it was easy enough to remember.

'Hi, Doc!'

'All right, Doc!'

One after the other they greeted me, stepping back to make room.

'Like yer perfume, Doc!' one prisoner said, sniffing the air.

I looked back over my shoulder. 'Thanks, it's Escape by Calvin Klein!'

The group loitering by the snooker table sniggered.

'Gimme some of that!' one of them shouted.

It had become a running joke at the Scrubs. A lot of the prisoners found it amusing when they discovered the name.

The nurse who was first on the scene had her back to us, blocking my view of the prisoner sitting on the treatment couch.

A sickening indefinable smell hung in the airless room. I swallowed hard to stop myself retching.

The nurse stepped to her right, revealing a truly shocking sight. Severe burns covered the man's naked body. His chest and both arms were blistered and bright red, with some areas oozing watery fluid, suggesting deep second-degree burns.

The prisoner was in his mid-forties and didn't even wince as the nurse applied another water-gel dressing. He wasn't speaking, just staring ahead with a glazed expression. He was in shock. Pale and sweating from the pain.

I pulled one of the nurses aside. 'Do we know his name?'

She shook her head.

'Do we know what happened?'

The nurse flashed me a look. A knowing glance I'd now seen on a number of occasions, when alluding to someone who was doing time for a sex crime.

'He was attacked by a gang while he was in the shower. They threw boiling sugar water over him.'

'For fuck's sake,' I whispered under my breath.

Sugar water was like acid in terms of the damage it caused to the skin. The prisoners used it because the effects were many times more painful and devastating than normal boiling water. The sugar glued to the skin, prolonging the time the burning water stayed in contact with the skin.

In all the years I worked in prisons, I never managed to come to terms with the sickening brutality I witnessed at times.

He was lucky the hot water hadn't hit his genitals, which was no doubt where the gang had been aiming. The burns along his arms were probably from where he had tried to protect himself.

My job was to prescribe strong painkillers for him, so that the nurses could give them to him without delay. Without a prescription they were not permitted to give anything stronger than paracetamol and ibuprofen.

'Thanks, Doc, we can handle this from here,' the nurse reassured me once I'd prescribed the drugs. 'The ambulance is on its way.'

I set off on the long walk back to Healthcare. It dawned on me that I might never see that man again. He would almost certainly be transferred to another prison for his own protection, and I hoped for his sake that wherever he went the prisoners would not find out what crime he had been sentenced for.

Chapter Fourteen

My heart was pounding as the security officers searched my bag. Even though I knew I had nothing to worry about, the random searches at the Scrubs were strangely intimidating.

Every member of staff arriving for work that day was directed into a part of the prison I never usually went to. We all had to put our bags through a scanner, and then line up to be checked by a sniffer dog before being rubbed down. If anything untoward was noted in the bags, we were taken to one side while they were checked.

They pulled out my essentials, one by one, placing them on the table. A Tupperware box with my lunch in it, a bottle of water, my purse with only a few pound coins in it – it was forbidden to take much money into the prison. The officer in charge unzipped the front pocket of my bag and stopped in his tracks. He glanced sideways at the other officer.

What had they found?

The officer furrowed his brow. 'What have we got here, then?'

'What?' I said, barely able to take the tension any more.

He removed a packet of chewing gum with only two pieces left in it, placing it on the table.

He leaned in towards me. 'You know you shouldn't have this?'

Chewing gum was on the list of things that should never be taken into the prison. I felt terrible, and deeply ashamed. I was also quite scared, feeling like a naughty school kid, worried that I could lose my job for breaking the rules.

I cringed. 'Yes, I do. I'm sorry.'

I hadn't realised it was in there as I wasn't using my normal bag that day. I'd been in London the day before, attending a course on substance misuse, and hadn't had time to decant everything back into my usual bag.

The security officer slid the gum across the table to his colleague.

'I'm afraid we are going to have to confiscate it,' he said, in a very formal tone.

'That's fine,' I replied, blushing with shame.

I scooped up my lunch from the table and threw it back in my oversized bag and made my way in as usual, minus my chewing gum.

I'd thought that would be the end of the matter, but just before my lunch break I was called in to see my boss. Karen was blonde, pretty, incredibly assertive and very good at her job as Associate Director for Central London Community Health.

CLCH ran various contracts, including one to provide medical care to the Scrubs. Technically, I was employed as a locum via an agency. Karen ran a very tight ship and didn't take any nonsense. I was surprised to find out my chewing gum mishap had made it back to her. I felt like I'd been called up in front of the headmistress, as she warned me about how potentially serious it could have been if a prisoner had got their hands on my gum!

I knew Karen was only doing her job and had to be sure that everyone working under her leadership understood and obeyed the rules without exception.

I apologised again, hoping that would finally be the end of the matter, but just after lunch she stuck her nose around the door of the doctors' office.

A feeling of dread filled my stomach.

'Amanda, would you mind popping in to see me,' she said, as she disappeared back into her office next door.

What had I done now? Was I in serious trouble? It couldn't be about the chewing gum again, could it? I was panicking as I made those few steps to see my boss.

I knocked on her door, waited for the invitation to 'Come in', and then entered.

To my horror, Governor Frake was standing next to Karen. It felt as if my stomach somersaulted twice over. It must be really serious to be summoned to see the head of Security.

I swallowed hard. 'If it's the chewing gum . . .' I started, but didn't get to finish my sentence as Governor Frake broke into a fit of violent coughs.

I suddenly realised I wasn't there because I was in trouble, I was there because I was a doctor.

'Amanda, would you mind taking a look at Vanessa? She's feeling very poorly.'

'Of course,' I said. 'I'll just pop next door to get my stethoscope'.

'I don't want to make a fuss,' Governor Frake said between coughs. 'I hate seeing doctors.'

I suspected that the governor wasn't the sort to take time off work, and that she would probably have to be on death's door before she finally called for help.

'It's just a little cough!' she said, spluttering all over the place. 'I've suffered from asthma for years.' She looked so unwell that I almost didn't need to listen to her chest to know she had a nasty infection.

She removed her black suit jacket, slinging it over the back of a chair, and lifted her shirt up so that I could listen to her chest. Her complexion was pale with a film of feverish sweat, and she looked utterly exhausted. She was short of breath and struggling to even complete a sentence.

I listened to her breathing. I felt strangely nervous in her presence as she was so formidable and I had so much respect for her.

'Deep breaths in and out through your mouth.'

The governor managed only half a breath before she erupted into a fit of coughing. Her chest sounded crackly and wheezy. I couldn't check her peak flow as I didn't have a meter with me, but she had all the signs of an acute infective exacerbation of her asthma.

I pulled the stethoscope from my ears, resting it around

my neck. She looked at me as if she knew what I was going to ask.

'Do you smoke?

She chortled. 'Name someone in here who doesn't. I know, I know, it's a bad habit, Doc, but it keeps me sane. I am trying to cut it down.'

She knew better than me that she needed to stop.

I wrote her a private prescription for antibiotics and steroids, and handed it across to her. She already had her inhalers.

For the first time since I'd started at the Scrubs, the governor cracked me a smile.

In her gravelly voice she said, 'Ta very much, Doc.'

At last I felt like Governor Frake approved of me, and accepted me as being worthy of working in the Scrubs, which made me feel surprisingly elated. I had sometimes sensed a divide between the prison staff and healthcare staff, as our roles were so different, so to feel accepted by someone I was in awe of was a good feeling.

'Are you going to take the rest of the day off, Vanessa?' Karen asked.

Governor Frake laughed.

'I'll be seeing you, ladies. Thanks again, Doc,' she said, and then disappeared out of the door. No doubt returning to patrolling the wings, rather than heading to her bed.

*

I set off for the Seg round after my consultation with the governor, as I had been too busy to go there in the morning.

When I arrived I found the BOSS chair back in residence again (Body Orifice Security Scanner). A large grey throne, it looked as if its purpose was to electrocute people, but it was actually a highly sensitive metal detector, designed to detect smuggled contraband.

'If we suspect a prisoner is concealing a phone or weapon up their arse,' Ed had told me, shortly after I'd started at the Scrubs, 'we sit them down on the BOSS chair. If it detects something, it makes a buzzing noise and a red light flashes on the back of the chair. Sometimes we turn the buzzer off and just rely on the flasher, so the prisoner won't know *we* know he's hiding something! He then has to stay in the Seg until he shits it out.'

The world I was working in was definitely not glamour ous!

My Seg round was punctuated with the usual mix of being ignored, being sworn at, and if I was lucky, an odd acknowledgement of thanks. That day, though, I was blown away by the lengths that one prisoner went to in order to say thank you.

Ed was leading me along the landing, thumping the cell doors, letting the inmates know I was there to help if they needed anything.

He banged his fist on the next cell. I knew the man inside, as he'd been on the Seg for a few weeks. He was in his fifties and had a history of violence, but had always been good with me. He'd been suffering from anxiety attacks while locked up in the Seg, but I'd been as supportive as possible, prescribing him medication to help.

'Doc's here!' Ed wrenched open the hatch, peered inside, and when he was reassured that the prisoner wasn't behaving threateningly, unlocked the door.

We stood in the doorway, staring into the gloom.

'How are you today?' I asked.

The man stepped forward into the light coming from the doorway.

He was stocky, bald, his skin creasing into folds around the back of his neck. He had a hooked nose, which looked like it had been broken a few times, and strikingly blonde eyebrows.

He held his left hand behind his back, awkwardly.

'I'm feeling better,' he said. 'Those pills helped a lot.'

'Is your left arm all right?'

The prisoner smiled shyly, showing just the tips of his teeth. He moved his concealed hand to the front, opening his fingers, one by one, to reveal a racing car, beautifully hand-carved out of his bar of soap.

'I made this for you, Doc,' he said, holding his palm out.

It was so touching and I couldn't quite believe he'd taken the time to painstakingly carve out the wheels, the steering wheel, the wing mirrors, all in the gloomy light of the Seg cell, for me. It was a little work of art.

'It's really beautiful, thank you so much,' I said. 'What have I done to deserve this?'

'It's for being kind and not judging me,' he replied.

I swallowed hard to get rid of the lump in my throat.

I carefully cupped the present in my hands, knowing then that it would be something I would always treasure.

I thanked him again before Ed locked the door.

I floated along the rest of the landing, on a high, reflecting on all the people I had met while working in prison – not just the inmates, but the inspirational colleagues I'd worked with along the way. The majority – by far – treated the prisoners fairly and professionally, doing their jobs to the best of their abilities. At times the treatment had to be harsh, but often kindness and compassion were evident. Only occasionally did I encounter someone whose behaviour was unkind and uncaring. One such person was a locum doctor who, thank goodness, had only worked in the Scrubs for about four months.

He was a bully who seemed to love the power his position offered. He appeared to hate the prisoners, showing them no compassion and treating them with utter contempt. He rarely prescribed any painkillers, and also tried to stop other doctors' prescriptions, even for something as simple as paracetamol.

The prisoners hated him, and a lot of the officers complained about his arrogant manner. We were all delighted when the news spread that he had left and was never coming back!

Ed broke my thoughts.

'You must be special, Doc,' he said. 'I don't get presents like that.'

*

I stirred my coffee, tapping the spoon on the rim, and placed the cup on the desk. I took a sip, the hot liquid scorching my mouth, but I was desperate for the caffeine hit before going down to Reception.

Haj announced that all the new arrivals were in, by the time I got to Reception, and that no more were expected that day.

'Many in?' I asked.

He grimaced. 'Afraid so.'

I logged on to my computer and braced myself for the next few hours in Reception.

At 8 p.m., as usual, we all trudged up to the FNC to continue seeing the new arrivals.

The first man that Haj showed into my room was nothing out of the ordinary. He was tall and thin, with an unhurried manner about him. He was wearing a rather moth-eaten, thick-knit fisherman's jumper, and generally appeared a bit unkempt.

He seemed so relaxed I wondered if he had been in and out of prison many times, as was so often the case, particularly with homeless people.

I didn't have any notes marked against his name, so his crime wasn't severe enough to warrant a warning from the nurses.

I began my list of questions, asking whether he was on remand or sentenced, whether he had a history of self-harm, any medical conditions, etc.

As I had suspected, Kai had been in prison before, but never in the Scrubs.

He leant back in his chair, yawning as he stretched his hands up behind his head. His face was expressionless, seemingly bored by having to speak to me.

'Any history of mental-health illness?' I went on.

He scratched his temple. 'I've been diagnosed with schizophrenia.'

'Are you on medication for that?'

He nodded. A glazed expression plastered across his face as if he'd had this conversation a thousand times before.

'Yep, Depixol.'

'And how have you been getting on with that?' I asked.

'Fine. Absolutely fine.' He yawned again, fanning his mouth with his hand. Was this feigned apathy? Was he simply trying to appear calm? Or was it a sign of something more?

Schizophrenia is not, as TV or cinema will often suggest, a case of a patient thinking they are two people. It's a far more complex mental illness, with a varied host of potential symptoms, including auditory and visual hallucinations, and an increased sense of detachment from reality.

Antipsychotic medications are used to control the disorder, and sometimes a combination of medication is needed. Patients are usually under the care of a psychiatrist, and the condition is manageable as long as they continue to take their medication.

I typed up my notes, Kai's eyes wandering around the room.

'How long have you been sentenced for?' I asked.

'Twelve weeks.'

'Not too bad then.'

He laughed half-heartedly.

My initial concerns about his behaviour seemed unfounded. He seemed well-adjusted to his medication, engaging well with me and answering my questions. All I needed to do was prescribe his medication and refer him to the psychiatrist.

But I could feel him staring at me as I finished writing up his notes, and I began to feel uneasy.

Suddenly he leapt out of his seat and started smashing his head against the wall! Whacking his head forcefully and repeatedly against the brickwork, my office filled with the awful sound of his skull reverberating against the brick.

'Stop!' I screamed.

But he kept going. Beating his head again and again. Narrowed eyes and gritted teeth. Staring at me, his hands clenched into fists. Did he mean to turn his anger on me?

I smacked my hand against the panic button to the left of my desk. Within seconds at least ten prison officers were charging into my room. He tried to fight them off – kicking, biting, throwing punches. Finally, they forced him to the ground and cuffed his arms behind his back. They lifted him up and carted him off. He wriggled and thrashed in their arms, his screams leaving a trail of echoes along the corridor.

Initially he was taken to a cell, and later that evening was admitted to Healthcare for observation, following the trauma to his head.

'Doc, are you all right?' Terry was there now. He touched my arm, concerned.

For a few seconds, the blood was pounding so loudly in my ears that I couldn't quite hear what he was saying.

'Doc? Doc? Are you okay?'

I shook my head trying to focus.

Suddenly I felt very self-conscious. It wasn't like me to call for help.

'I'm sorry for making a fuss!' I said, trying to appear unruffled.

'It's okay to be afraid,' Terry reassured me. 'That was the right thing to do. He could've come at you.'

Which was true, and I'd feared as much. But I'd acted for the prisoner's own safety too. 'He was hitting his head so hard, I was scared he was going to fracture his skull.'

I began to shake with relief. In a matter of seconds, the support system around me had been proven, all of us working together to keep everyone safe. Still, as much as I liked to think I was tough, that was the first time since working in prison I had felt fear. Real fear. Fear for my life.

My fingers were trembling as I finished writing up my notes on Kai.

Haj popped in to see if I was okay.

I was. It was over, and the shift went on. There were still many more men waiting to be seen. The work didn't care how afraid you were, it still demanded to be done.

Chapter Fifteen

If asked, David would have agreed that my language had gone downhill.

It was hard not to pick up swear words when that was pretty much all I heard in the Scrubs. Luckily, he is very understanding, and decided not to pass comment at the string of expletives I fired at the lady in the Aston Martin behind, who was hooting impatiently at me to pull out into oncoming traffic.

'Deep breath,' David advised instead, in his soft Yorkshire accent.

I was feeling increasingly unforgiving towards the residents of my wealthy neighbourhood, and, strangely, more kindly disposed to the prisoners I was meeting. Something was shifting in me. The people I was caring for in the prison felt more real. Their lives, the struggles they faced, their extraordinary stories were far more interesting than the sort of conversations I used to have at local drinks parties.

My language and my mood were just as bad the following day, when I was coming to the end of a shift in the First Night Centre. By that point, I'd lost count of the number of evenings

I'd welcomed prisoners into the Scrubs. *I've been here long enough to work this computer system with my eyes shut,* I thought, staring daggers at the frozen screen.

'Oh for fuck's sake,' I hissed at the computer.

I looked bashfully at the prisoner sitting in the chair next to me. 'Sorry!'

'What have you got to be sorry for?' he said. He was a homeless man who only had a few front teeth left. 'What do I care if you swear?'

I had met him now on quite a few occasions, and always found him to be a quiet, gentle man. We had almost become friends. However, I was taken aback when he said, 'It's good to see you again, Doctor Brown. It's like meeting an angel in a shit-hole.'

I couldn't help giggling and he smiled back. I think it was one of the nicest compliments anyone had ever paid me!

'Thanks, mate,' I said.

I still had a smile on my face when the next prisoner walked into my room. But that was quickly wiped off when I saw who I was about to deal with.

The man stared at me stonily. His hands were deep in his jean pockets, his features screwed up into a sneer.

I shuddered. After Kai I was a bit more on edge about prisoners who looked threatening or intimidating.

I smiled to try to defuse the tension.

'Would you like to take a seat?' I pointed to the chair next to me.

He had a skinhead, and tattoos creeping up his neck. He

rolled up his sleeves to his elbows, revealing a multitude more tattoos. He was probably in his early thirties. White. Average height and build.

I was feeling increasingly uncomfortable but tried to appear relaxed.

He slumped into the chair. Crossing his arms, he glared at me, a look on his face that was almost loathing.

From the nurses' notes I could see that his name was Ian, and the only medication he needed prescribing were inhalers for his asthma.

I started typing, sorting out his inhalers and going through the other routine questions. I'd come to learn that a lot of the prisoners who present with anger are often masking hurt. As always, I resolved to try to understand rather than to simply fear, to try to offer more support than a simple prescription.

I asked Ian about his support network. Did he have anyone on the outside who cared about him?

'I got a girlfriend. A kid,' he said, his voice flat.

'How old is your child?'

'Mia, she's three.'

He started relaxing a little, the scowl lifting from his brow.

'You must miss them?'

'Yeah, it's hard on all of us when I'm inside.'

'Will they come and visit you? How long are you here for?'

'Five months.' He then cracked a hint of a smile at the

thought of his partner and Mia. 'I hope, so, they promised they would.'

I was relieved that he was gently relaxing and opening up to me.

I glanced at my notes. 'Have you always lived in Acton?'

'Nah, I grew up in Sunderland. In a care home.'

'That's sad. Did you ever know your parents?'

Ian uncrossed his arms and rubbed his eyes, forcefully.

'My real mum, she got in touch recently. For the first time.'

I felt a surge of happiness for a man who was a virtual stranger.

'So you'll see her?'

He kicked the leg of my desk with his trainer.

'Nah, I'm not interested. I've got no intention of meeting her.'

He shifted in his chair. Ian was clearly feeling increasingly uncomfortable, and I was feeling increasingly sorry for him.

'That's such a shame, why do you feel that way?'

An uncomfortable silence hung in the air. He stared at the ground, chewing on his thoughts. Finally, he lifted his gaze to me, his eyes heavy with sorrow.

'Because I'm afraid of being rejected again.'

It was late at night and I was exhausted. Ian's story touched me. Suddenly the feelings of loss, sadness and helplessness overwhelmed me and I could feel myself welling up. I couldn't help but think how horrific it would be if I never saw my boys again. My heart went out to Ian's mother. God knows what might have led her to give up her child all those years ago. I somehow wanted to help her as much as I wanted to help Ian.

I thought about Jared at Huntercombe Prison. How he too had grown up in a care home, and would have longed to hear from his mum.

It was such a wonderful opportunity for Ian to heal some of the scars from the past. I wasn't naïve enough to think everything would be rosy if Ian did meet his mum; she might have a lot of problems herself. But I could see how much he was hurting, and yearning for answers to questions which may have been plaguing him for years.

Cautiously, I suggested, 'As a mother myself, I'd guess she's probably longing to hear from you. Maybe it's worth the risk of rejection?'

Finally, my emotions took over and silent tears pooled in my eyes. Ian must have sensed the power of a mother's love, and it seemed to flick a switch in him. The young man, who on first impressions had appeared so intimidating and angry, sensed my sadness, and in a total role reversal, he reached out to comfort me.

He gave me a big, caring hug.

I dabbed my eyes dry. His face appeared so gentle, and he looked at me with such kindness.

He didn't say another word as he turned to leave, but I was sure a lot of conflicting feelings and emotions were churning around in his head.

'Ian.' I stopped him at the door. 'Good luck with every-thing.'

All signs of aggression had now evaporated. He gave me a beautiful smile.

*

When I had finished seeing Ian it was 10 p.m. and time to go home.

Haj and I walked out together from the FNC, along the fourth floor landing on B Wing, and down the endless metal stairs to the exit gates.

Sharing the gates was always quicker with two people.

Haj had to go and get something from his locker, so I continued on my own past the seemingly never-ending rows of small windows of the four floors of B Wing, with the magnificent chapel to my left, towards the gatehouse.

Sometimes prisoners would shout out, 'Night, Doc', or 'Night, miss', with an occasional, 'God bless ya.'

I never really knew which window the greeting came from, but it always gave me a little glow of happiness and reinforced my feeling of belonging.

Sadly, there were no such greetings that night. My shoulders were hunched forward with the weight of the day. I pulled my coat tightly round me, as the wind was bitingly cold. As I walked past the last few cells of the Seg, at the far end of B Wing, a deep voiced blasted out 'Piss off home, you old cunt. I hope you get run over by a bus on the way.'

I didn't look up, but kept on walking.

I was almost too tired to care, and felt drained of all my emotions. The day had been hard and I was longing to get home – but the prisoner's hurtful words rattled around in my head.

Soon I would be past the imposing building and at the gatehouse.

There was always a feeling of relief, to get beyond the prison walls and the endless rows of windows with unknown eyes watching.

It was not uncommon for things to be thrown at whoever may be walking by. One nurse was hit by an orange; one of the doctors had a curry tipped over him.

No doubt it was good sport for the prisoners, but there was always the worry of a direct hit by something or other.

My only near miss had been when I was walking outside with one of the nurses, past C Wing, and water was thrown at us – we hoped it was water and not urine! We walked on quicker, not daring to look up.

I wasn't in the mood to play dodge that night.

The night air was cold and damp. My breath steamed up into the sky as I stared ahead at the forbidding walls. One more gate and I would be in the courtyard leading to the gatehouse.

I handed my keys in to the officer on duty, clipped my tally on the chain, and wished him a good night.

'See you tomorrow, Doc', he said, his voice fading as the solid iron door slid shut behind me.

I closed my eyes and inhaled a big gulp of air. Holding the cold in my lungs for a few moments before sighing it out, along with all the crap of the day.

*

I wedged the pillows behind my back, picked up my mug of weak tea and drank it, enjoying the wonderful relief of being tucked up in bed. David had drifted off to sleep beside me.

I opened the book by my bedside, hoping the last few pages of the chapter would be enough to lull me to sleep. It worked, my eyes quickly growing tired. Blindly, I turned off my bedside light and settled down to sleep.

But my body had tricked me. It was just after 2 a.m. when I woke with a start, and in the quiet of the night my brain just wouldn't settle.

I thought of the prisoners in the Seg, staring up at the ceiling. With no end in sight, the days and nights must have felt like an eternity.

I was desperate for sleep. I was so tired, and had to get up again at 4.30, but I was wide awake. All my problems became magnified as I lay there restlessly under the sheets. I started to question what I was doing with my life. Why was I working so hard, only to be told by someone who I was there to help that they wished me dead? Was I making any difference to any of the prisoners, or was it all just a waste of time? I hated the idea of quitting, but wondered if it was time.

David stirred and rolled over. I felt jealous of how peacefully he slept. If my body hadn't been so achy, I would have crept downstairs to the study and tipped all of my anger out onto a blank page on the computer – although I'd become slightly wary of doing that when I was emotional; last time it had landed me on the cover of a magazine.

Instead, I rolled over onto my side and eventually managed to drift off.

I felt surprisingly robust when I woke an hour or so later.

I'd gone to bed feeling worthless, but had woken up determined not to be beaten by the day before's hurtful words.

I closed the front door quietly behind me, so as not to wake my family, walking briskly to the car in the chilly morning air. I turned on the ignition, the heating, and watched the exhaust billowing into the air in my rear-view mirror. I felt surprisingly calm and positive. With a forty-minute journey into London, I had plenty of time to prepare what I was going to say, and had worked out which cell the abuse was likely to have come from.

Chapter Sixteen

I walked confidently up to the door and nodded to Ed to give him the go ahead.

Bang. Bang. 'Doc's here,' he announced.

'Not interested,' came the reply.

No doubt about it, it was definitely him. The harsh tone. The same loud voice, hoarse from cigarettes.

I had suspected it was him, as the shouting had come from his direction, but his reply had confirmed it.

The man in question was big, his clothes stretched, his bed creaking under him. He was serving life for murder, and was awaiting transfer to a Cat A prison. They'd put him on the Seg as he was deemed too dangerous to be anywhere else.

I had seen him on a few occasions, and he had always been relatively polite to me, which was why I felt doubly hurt by his tirade of abuse.

Ed turned the key in the lock and opened the door.

I glared at the prisoner.

'Why did say you hoped I'd get run over by a bus last night?' I asked.

I held his gaze, not looking away, determined not to be intimidated. As it was, he didn't challenge me, his face immediately dropping to his chest, his words quiet.

'That was you?' he mumbled. 'I'm so sorry, Doc, I didn't know. I just shout out at anyone at night to relieve the boredom.'

He looked ashamed and a bit sheepish.

'Well, it was really hurtful, but thank you for apologising,' I said, inwardly feeling a huge sense of achievement for standing up for myself. I remembered the advice I'd received when I'd first started working at the Scrubs: to walk with confidence, to show authority. This was the same thing: not letting a prisoner walk all over me.

I softened slightly. 'While I'm here, is there anything you need to see me about?'

'No thanks,' he said, still looking at the floor, clearly embarrassed.

'Okay then, see you tomorrow.'

Ed slammed the cell door shut.

'Feel better?' he asked.

'Much!' I replied, grinning.

Five years in the Scrubs may have pushed me to the edge at times, but it had helped me to find my voice. I was beginning to feel more confident and assertive.

On the other hand, I certainly hadn't become immune to seeing pain and suffering. I doubted I ever would. However tough I thought I had become, I couldn't ever quite control my emotions when confronted by it.

I don't think I've ever felt so overwhelmed with pity as I did on one cold winter's night in Reception.

I was just wrapping things up, getting ready to go upstairs to the FNC, when Haj popped his head around the door. There was a look on his face, something had clearly disturbed him.

'I've got one more for you, Doc.' He stepped inside my room, closing the door behind him. He lowered his voice.

'Apparently, he sustained serious injuries after jumping out of a window on the third floor of a block of flats. He was trying to escape from the police. He's in a wheelchair, and has just been discharged from hospital, so it would be easier to see him down here.'

'OK,' I said, switching my computer back on and entering my password. I was looking at my screen when Haj returned, pushing a man in a wheelchair.

I turned round and, to my horror, the injuries were far worse than I had anticipated. Both the prisoner's legs had been amputated, with just two small stumps remaining.

The man, who was in his thirties, looked petrified. His eyes were as wide as saucers. His hands were trembling. Sheer panic was etched on his face. All I wanted to do was reach out and comfort him. But he couldn't understand me as he didn't speak a word of English.

I tried anyway, hoping my voice and smile could soothe him.

'Please don't be frightened,' I said.

I looked down at his stumps, which were wrapped in

bandages from the recent surgery. His injuries must have been extremely severe for him to have had his legs amputated just below hip level. They must have shattered to pieces in the fall.

His whole life had been turned upside down. He hadn't just been stripped of his freedom, he also had to come to terms with the loss of both legs. I couldn't imagine how terrified he must feel, being locked up in a vast, intimidating prison, unable to understand a word anyone was saying, or to tell anyone if he was in pain. Trying to absorb the reality of his horrific injuries must have been devastating.

Normally I would have phoned Language Line for an interpreter, but there wasn't enough time. It was already 8 p.m. and the officers and the rest of the new inmates were being moved up to the FNC.

The details of the man's full story would be sorted out the following morning with the help of the interpreting service. For that night, I just needed to make sure that he was safe, not in pain, and that someone would be on hand to help him with his physical needs, such as going to the toilet, and getting in and out of his bed. He would definitely need to be located in a disabled cell, but I was worried that there might not be one free, as there were only a few available. I phoned Healthcare but, unusually, there was no answer.

I was becoming increasingly concerned as, apart from one officer, Haj and I and the new inmate were the only people left in the dark and dingy Reception. I asked Haj to try to contact the duty governor, and while I waited I prescribed the same strong painkillers that the inmate had been given in hospital. I would not normally prescribe opiate-based analgesia, as they can be highly addictive and used as 'currency' within the prison, but this was obviously a special circumstance. The man was likely to be in a lot of pain for some time.

He sat there quietly, in his wheelchair, staring into space. I wished I could speak to him and break his trance, but I knew it was futile.

I heard footsteps outside and then a looming figure appeared in my doorway.

'Doctor Brown.'

It was Shiny Shoes.

I stood up. 'Thank you for coming to see me, there's something I need to discuss with you.'

The governor nodded. 'Go on,' he said.

'If you don't mind?' I indicated I'd rather continue the conversation out of earshot of the prisoner. He may not have been able to understand what we were saying, but a sense of respect, alone, made me uncomfortable discussing his needs in front of him.

An officer stepped in to man the door, while I walked to the end of the corridor with Shiny Shoes. I was feeling angry and frustrated that the inmate had been discharged from hospital to prison so late in the day, and with no advanced warning so that we could prepare a suitable cell for him.

His surgery was certainly far too recent for him to have

had prosthetic limbs fitted, and he would need assistance with his daily care. I explained to Shiny Shoes that I could not get an answer from Healthcare, and needed his help to make sure that the prisoner would be located in a suitable cell.

Shiny Shoes rubbed his eyes with his forefinger and thumb. He'd clearly had as draining a day as I had. He sighed deeply.

'We definitely have to find a disabled cell for him. I'll sort it out. Somehow.'

He could see that I was getting increasingly upset.

'Doctor Brown,' he said, 'you mustn't let it get to you.'

I said the only words that I could find, which to this day I still truly believe.

'The day I lose compassion is the day I will stop working. I'm afraid it will *always* get to me.'

He smiled gently, and I knew he understood.

But of course he had the correct attitude for running a prison. These men were criminals who were being punished for their crimes, and he couldn't afford to get sentimental. I understood that. But I would never be able to become like that. If I did, I would lose who I was as a person.

Shiny Shoes contacted Healthcare and managed to organise a suitable cell. Haj and the officer wheeled the inmate away.

'Let me know if you need anything else,' Shiny Shoes said. He checked his watch and his expression switched. His thoughts were already somewhere else – working on another problem in another part of the prison, no doubt.

Finally, I was alone in the dark and gloomy room, except for a little mouse that went scuttling by. I felt exhausted and worn down with sadness, and I sat down, held my head in my hands, and sobbed, and sobbed, and sobbed. For so many people, for so many sadnesses, and tonight especially for the tragedy of that young man.

Chapter Seventeen

Being called to an attempted suicide was, sadly, not unusual. Everyone dreaded hearing the Code Blue call. As I raced along the long corridors to C Wing, I had no idea if I was going to be too late. Officers and nurses were also running from different directions to the same location.

Every year I attended a refresher course in Intermediate Life Support, because it was so commonly needed in prisons, and I was always grateful for the annual update.

There wasn't much of a crowd gathered on the landing outside the cell, so I presumed that the poor man had only just been found.

When I arrived, out of breath, I was relieved to find that a doctor I had never met before was already there, applying chest compressions. He looked up at me through his dark floppy hair, which was clumped together with sweat. CPR was hard work, which is why it was usually necessary to take it in turns.

'Thank God you're here,' he said.

I dropped to my knees beside the prisoner, ready to take over. The cell seemed smaller than most, although it probably only felt that way. The young doctor shuffled around one to where a nurse had been crouched, giving the man oxygen via the Ambubag. The nurse rose to his feet, retreating to the doorway.

'Don't stand there,' the young doctor said. 'You're blocking the bloody light.'

Tempers were frayed, although that was no excuse for rudeness.

I missed my friend Zaid, and our lunch breaks watching the rats. He'd had enough of the politics going on between the Security and the Healthcare departments. Frustrated with the difficulty of getting patients to their hospital appointments, he'd decided to stop working at the Scrubs, which had saddened me.

Zaid wouldn't have lost his temper, I thought, as I crossed my hands and started pumping the man's chest.

One, two, three . . .

I wondered why the man had tried to hang himself.

Four, five, six . . .

He was a white man, I guessed in his mid-fifties. His neck showed angry red ligature marks from his strangulation.

Seven, eight, nine . . .

'How long has he been like this?' I asked.

The new doctor grimaced. 'Over five minutes.'

'Oh!' I puffed, between compressions, worried about how long the inmate might have been starved of oxygen. I kept pumping, and counting. Every thirty compressions, the doctor would give the man two bursts of oxygen from the air bag. Thankfully, reinforcements arrived very quickly with the defibrillator, and the pads were applied to his chest. An officer had already ripped the inmate's T-shirt open to get access. The machine's robotic voice said, 'Shock required; Shock now; Shock.'

'Clear!' shouted the new doctor. I slid back quickly, the metal of the bed frame digging into my back.

The prisoner's body convulsed into the air as the doctor pressed the shock button.

My heart was racing as we continued our resuscitation attempt until, thank God, the paramedics arrived.

By then several officers and two more nurses, including Sylvie, had appeared.

As the paramedics carried the prisoner off to the ambulance, a stunned silence hung in the cell as we digested the drama of the last ten minutes and the relief that we had managed to keep him alive.

I rose to my feet, shaking the blood back into my legs, and made my way over to where Sylvie was leaning over the railings. I joined her, resting my forearms on the metal. She glanced at me sideways, sympathetically, not saying a word. She may not have seen the worst of it, but she didn't have to. We all knew what it was like to be called out to an attempted suicide.

When she finally spoke, the words were music to my ears. 'Fancy a cuppa?'

'I'd love one' I replied instantly.

Before we traipsed back to the nurses' common room,

I turned to one of the nearby officers. 'Any idea who he is, or anything about him?'

He shook his head. 'The only thing I do know is that he was recently given a twelve-year sentence.'

I supposed that he had just shown us how he felt about that. About how capable he felt of being trapped in the Scrubs for that amount of time.

Sylvie and I walked back together in silence, deep in thought.

I wondered how it must feel to face the prospect of spending years in prison, and how desperate that man – who none of us knew – must have felt to try to escape, the only way he could.

Chapter Eighteen

I craved a walk in the fields behind my house. I felt in great need of a dose of nature to soothe away the brutality of the past months – to bring me back into a gentle place, far away from the violence and the noise.

Walking was the therapy I needed to prevent myself from becoming traumatised by all the distressing things I was witnessing on a daily basis.

Working in a prison could be grim, depressing and draining. Reconnecting with the beauty of the world was a tonic for me, an even more important part of my life than it had been before.

As I made my way along the woodland path, the words of one of my favourite poems floated into my head:

What is this life if, full of care,
We have no time to stand and stare?

I had learnt William Henry Davies' *Leisure* off by heart when I was a child, and the meaning has never faded from my mind.

I stopped in my tracks, alone in the woods, listening intently to the woodland creatures. The birds, the rustling, the sound of the fallen leaves being swept along by the autumn breeze.

I craned my head to the sky, staring through the canopy at the fluffy white clouds, morphing into different shapes as they sailed past, the words of the poem on my lips.

The world isn't so bad after all, I smiled to myself.

And its beauty should never be taken for granted. Day in, day out, I was surrounded by people who were stripped of their freedom, who would have done anything to be standing where I was then, taking pleasure in the simple things in life.

All I needed to do was step out of my back door to see greenery. Some of the prisoners I was dealing with would have to wait five, ten, fifteen years to have that pleasure. Some might never be able to walk through a woodland again. The best view they would ever have was of the sky from the exercise yard.

I drew in a deep breath, taking the nature deep into my lungs.

I walked on, thinking about the man who lost his legs, about Azar who struggled so much to adjust, of Jared the teenager I'd met all those years ago. Those people, and many more, stayed with me on my walks. They all, in their different ways, had enriched my life and made me appreciate everything that I had, especially my wonderful family. They had taught me to never envy anyone their wealth or possessions, nor to take my freedom for granted.

At times such thoughts could have brought me to tears, but the words of the poem were making me feel happy and rejuvenated.

I was free, I was healthy, I had everything to live for.

The light grew brighter as I neared the edge of the woodland. The tunnel of trees opened into a paddock, forcing me to squint into the glorious autumn sun. The sweet aroma of the ripe blackberries woven through the hedgerows wafted in my direction.

I stood and stared. A simple forty-five-minute walk had restored my equilibrium, and I felt calm and at peace with the world. I also felt hopeful and positive about my work and that maybe, just occasionally, I could make a difference.

*

My positive thoughts were brought to life the next day while I was walking through B Wing on my way to Healthcare.

The prisoners were out in force, milling around for association hour. When I first started working at the Scrubs I was warned that it wasn't safe for me to walk through the wings during association time, nor between the wings during free flow, which is when large groups of prisoners are escorted by officers to different areas of the prison, perhaps to attend education or to go to and from their places of work.

But I wasn't the slightest bit afraid. I felt like I was part of the furniture. Often the prisoners would stop to shake my hand, say hello, tell me how their day was going, have a moan about something or other, and sometimes we would have a good laugh, as some of their humour was wonderful. I enjoyed the interaction, as it made me feel that I belonged there and was no longer an outsider.

As I passed the pool table, a loud voice from above cut across the chatter.

'Doc, Doc!'

I swivelled around and looked up.

The man was leaning over the landing watching the world go by, his arms casually resting on the railing.

He smiled broadly.

'Hi, Doc, do you remember me?'

I recognised him instantly. His story had stayed with me ever since we'd met.

He tried to say something but his words were lost in the noise – the talking, the shouting, the sound of the pool balls smacking against each other, the high ceilings amplifying every little sound.

He held his hand up. 'Wait a minute, I'm coming down.'

The man flew down the metal stairs at lightning speed, eager to catch up with me.

I greeted him with a warm smile; I was just as happy to see him as he was to see me. We'd only met once, but the feelings he'd invoked had stayed with me.

Slightly out of breath, he puffed, 'I've been hoping to run into you.'

His expression was a far cry from the angry, embittered

one that he had worn as he walked into my room all those weeks ago. He looked positively ecstatic.

'How are you, Ian?' I asked.

He could hardly contain his happiness. His glacial blue eyes were sparkling with joy, a rare thing to see in the Scrubs.

'I've contacted my mum!'

I was stunned into silence. Not in a million years did I think Ian would have accepted his mother's olive branch of reconciliation. He had seemed so angry, so bitter about being abandoned and left to grow up in a care home, that I thought there was no chance of him changing his mind. Perhaps my words had hit home?

He looked at me intensely. 'You were right, Doc. It was worth the risk. My mum is coming to visit me this weekend.'

And then his whole expression seemed to melt, and his eyes sparkled with happiness as he announced, 'We're going to be a family again.'

I really wanted to give him the biggest hug, but didn't dare to in the middle of the wing.

That magical moment confirmed how it's often the simple things you do for people, things you almost forget as the day whizzes by, that can make the biggest difference. Those few encouraging words I had said to Ian when we first met may have changed his life for ever. I would love to think so.

Having family was usually one of the most important things for the prisoners. Someone to care about them, visit them, wait for them, help them to get back on their feet when they were released. It was often the driving force that helped them cope with being banged up.

It may not have been medicine, but I felt that I had helped heal Ian in a different way. He in turn had made me feel good about the job I was doing. Perhaps it was all worthwhile, and that actually caring that little bit more really was making a difference to some people.

'Cherish that time with your mum. I hope it all works out. I would love to know how it goes,' I said, before continuing on my way.

I would have really loved to hear about the reunion with his mum, but the chances were that I would probably never see him again. Some prisoners left my life as quickly as they had entered it. I could only hope that I may have helped a few of them in some way on their journey.

*

There was one prison visitor that never seemed to leave. Most of the time we rubbed along together quite nicely, never getting in each other's way. But as with all good relationships, there is often a tipping point, as I discovered on my lunch break one day.

For some time, I'd been sneaking off to have a nap in my lunch hour. I followed the same ritual I used in the mornings – unrolling my sleeping bag across three rather grimy-looking chairs, in one of the quiet therapy rooms in the Seacole Centre. Surprisingly, I'd only been disturbed once in the seven years I'd been working at the Scrubs. The nurse must have thought I was a dead body at first. 'Oh it's you, Doctor Brown!' she'd exclaimed, and then left me to it. Within seconds I had fallen back to sleep, I was so tired.

There was one secret ingredient that helped me fall asleep even faster though. Aside from my pillow and my sleeping bag, I always kept a bar of my favourite milk chocolate in my bag.

As I lay snuggled inside my cocoon, my head resting on my travel pillow, I would pull my eye mask down and blindly reach my hand down into my bag and break off a single square of chocolate.

The sensation of it melting in my mouth . . . the heavenly sweet taste . . . and I was asleep within seconds.

Today was no different. The chocolate melted.

I drifted off.

Totally refreshed when I woke, I decided to check on the chocolate – to ensure adequate supplies remained. To my horror, as well as the chocolate I discovered a scattering of mouse droppings in my bag – and they weren't just *in the bag*, they were also *inside the opened wrapper!* I realised that I had almost certainly eaten some with my chocolate! I felt disgusted. I took the bag and all its contents home with me that night, washed everything, and from that day on all consumables were kept in a tightly sealed plastic container!

I blamed myself. I had been stupid to think they wouldn't have crept into my bag at night for a nibble, as mice were all over the prison.

Not long after that a prisoner on E Wing was moaning to me that he had a Creme Egg on his shelf, that he was saving for a treat, but was dismayed when he woke in the night to find a mouse happily chomping away at it.

I felt for him!

*

The medicine I was practising at the Scrubs was very different from how I'd worked at my old GP practice. Working in the prison felt like firefighting, dealing with one crisis after another. I loved the drama and the excitement, but there was a part of me that was missing the problem-solving side of medicine. So when I was asked to see a young man who was very unwell, I embraced the challenge.

The prisoner staggered into the room, shivering and sweating.

He was a tall, sinewy Somalian man, who I could see from his notes had been transferred from another prison two days previously.

I instinctively went to his side to support him, as he was so unsteady on his feet, and gently helped him onto the couch.

I introduced myself, and asked him to tell me about his symptoms. He just stared through me with a glazed expression, and was unable to answer.

I saw from his notes that he was 23 years of age.

Sylvie had asked me to see him as she was so concerned about him.

'How long has he been like this?'

She shrugged. 'Since he arrived, but we don't know how long he was unwell before he transferred, as there aren't many notes on him.'

Abdi lay on the couch, and was shaking and sweating. He had a high temperature. Eventually he started to engage and answer my questions. He said that he had a very severe headache, and had been vomiting, and that for the past few weeks he had been feeling tired and non-specifically unwell, and had had a cough.

He had mild neck stiffness but no rash. I then checked his eye movements, and noted that he had nystagmus – an involuntary movement of his eyes. He also flinched away when I pointed a light in his eyes, indicating photophobia. Clearly he was desperately unwell, and needed urgent hospital admission.

I knew, as always, that I would have a battle on my hands to arrange for his admission to hospital. Abdi remained lying on the couch. He was so tall that his long skinny legs were dangling off the end.

Just as I had finished assessing him, the senior officer in charge of C Wing came in to see me. I hadn't met him before, although I was sure I'd heard his thick Geordie accent echoing across the wing when I was passing through.

'What's going on 'ere, Doc?' he said, his hands on his hips. 'Our Sylvie says you might be wantin' us to take him to hospital.' He nodded at Abdi.

I was sick and tired of putting up a fight for what I believed to be the right thing.

'He needs urgent medical attention and has to be admitted *today*! I suspect that he has a serious infection affecting his nervous system, and likely needs intravenous antibiotics.'

I glanced across to Abdi, but he was so out of it he didn't even react to what I'd said. I was glad, in a way. I didn't want to alarm him. However, I knew I had to put a strong case across to get him admitted to hospital.

The officer rolled back onto his heels, laughing. 'Get away, man, ye joking?' he scoffed. Tapping his watch, he said, 'It's 5 p.m., can't it wait until we have more officers to cover? He'll be all right until the mornin', Doc.'

I was furious! Incensed that someone with no medical training at all should make such a comment!

I was feeling strong, angry and determined. After all the fights I'd had to put up over the years, I was no longer intimidated by the prison officers, whatever their rank.

I mirrored the officer's hands-on-hips look, and almost hissed the words, 'He's got to go in tonight.'

Whatever venom I injected into my voice worked. 'Whatever you say, Doc,' the officer said, and with that he radioed Oscar One, to arrange the ambulance.

I returned to Abdi's side.

'Well done,' Sylvie said. 'I know it's not easy sometimes.'

She looked down at Abdi, who was floating in and out of consciousness.

'Are you okay to stay with him?' I asked Sylvie. 'I need to be in Reception.'

'Go, go.' She waved me off. 'Of course I'll stay with him.'

I was feeling particularly victorious about pushing for what I needed, when I heard my name echo across C Wing. There was only one woman in the whole of the prison who had a set of lungs on her like that.

'Hello!' I greeted Governor Frake, my voice rising an octave from nerves. She waited for me to draw closer. It was ridiculous that I was still intimidated by her presence, but I couldn't help it.

'Hello, Doctor Brown,' she said. 'I want a word with you.'

Chapter Nineteen

'Doc,' Frake said, almost shyly, 'I've got a favour to ask.'

I wondered what on earth the head of Security would need my help with.

She lowered her voice. 'I've been awarded an MBE.'

'Oh, that's wonderful news! Congratulations!' I was truly delighted for her, and not the slightest bit surprised. Governor Frake had turned the Scrubs into one of the most secure prisons in the UK, and for a woman to work her way up to such a high position, in a predominantly man's world, as it was back then, was a great achievement and definitely worthy of such recognition.

I was thrilled and full of admiration for her.

'Thanks,' she replied. 'It's just I've got nothing to wear to meet the Queen! I don't own a single dress, never have. I look ridiculous in them. So I'm going to need a smart suit, but have no idea where to buy one.' She looked especially sheepish. 'I just wondered if you might know where to try.'

I was taken aback. The thought of going shopping with the mighty governor was a bit surreal!

'You always look smart and professional, and I thought you would be the best person to ask for advice!' she said.

'Of course I'll help!' I said, ridiculously excited at the prospect.

It was a slow process, but little by little I was feeling accepted as one of the overall team, rather than just as one of the doctors.

But this came at a cost. Bit by bit I was also feeling more estranged from the world I lived in.

*

Every summer, an ex-colleague of mine called Peter held a magnificent garden party in the grounds of his beautiful house in Bucklebury.

He was a very successful orthopaedic surgeon, whom I had known for many years. We had first met in 1980 when we were doing our surgical house jobs together.

Anyone who was anyone in the community was invited, as well as many of his current and ex-colleagues. It was a chance to exchange stories and, for a cringe-inducing few, the opportunity to brag about money or how well their children were doing.

It was a beautiful day, and I should have been excited about the change of scene from the grime of the prison. But for some reason I was feeling apprehensive as David and I pulled into the car park in the paddock.

'What's that face for?' David asked.

I sighed. 'I feel exhausted and can't be bothered to make an effort.'

'Come on, we don't have to stay long,' he said.

Peter was a good friend, and I really appreciated the fact that he invited us to his party every year. He always made me feel welcome, despite the fact that my job was definitely not as glamorous, nor as prestigious, as those of most of the other guests. A lot of people simply couldn't understand why I would want to surround myself with criminals when I could still be working as a community GP. They struggled to see the value in what I was doing, and I found that upsetting and hurtful.

I ruffled my hand through my hair, painted on a smile, and patted David on the knee, indicating that I was ready to enter a different sort of fray.

The lawn was full of familiar faces, a kaleidoscope of colour and stunning designer outfits.

I looped arms with David, and we made a beeline towards Peter, who was standing next to the champagne glass tower.

He gave us a friendly wave and beckoned us over.

I felt incredibly uncomfortable – a fish out of water – which was bizarre considering I'd spent decades mingling with these folk.

I grabbed a glass of champagne from a passing waiter, and knocked half of it back. The fizz stung my dry throat.

'What do you have to do to get a pint around here?' David mumbled. He was not one for champagne.

A very tall man suddenly appeared in front of us.

'Amanda!' he said enthusiastically.

I recognised his face, but couldn't quite remember his name. Luckily, he saved me the embarrassment.

'Graham,' he said, holding his hand out to shake David's.

I'd met Graham at Peter's previous summer party; he was professor of something or other at a nearby teaching hospital.

I smiled, politely. 'Lovely to see you again.'

Before either David or I could say anything, Graham began telling us all about his children. A daughter who had read Economics at Oxford and was now working in the city; a son with a first-class honours degree in . . .

My mind wandered off. I began to feel slightly queasy. I really didn't belong there.

David bravely interrupted Graham with a comment about Wimbledon, only to have Graham bring the conversation back around to himself.

'Ah yes,' he said, throwing his head back and laughing. 'I used to play tennis for the first team at Guy's, back in the good old student days!'

I really couldn't stomach much more of this.

We managed to sidle away from Graham, and David found some friends that he'd been sailing with . . . but I felt strangely empty and lonely as I realised that I simply didn't belong in this world any more. More importantly, I didn't want to. I just wanted to go home.

I whispered into David's ear, 'I can't be doing with this any more.'

My values were changing, and my heart was clearly in another place. This old life felt shallow and empty.

*

'Is this your first time in prison?' I asked, making my way down the list of questions I asked all the new prisoners.

It was late, close to 10 p.m. Everyone looked tired, but David West's weathered appearance told another story.

'Yes,' he replied, calmly.

So calmly. I glanced up from my screen.

He immediately struck me as different.

He was casually dressed, with messy, sandy-coloured hair, unshaven. At a glance he looked like many of the homeless people I had met, but his demeanour was one of a man of wealth.

He was unnaturally calm for someone who hadn't been in prison before. I wondered if he was in shock, but as I looked into his grey-blue eyes I didn't see fear or panic. If I wasn't mistaken, I saw relief.

I felt compelled to find out more about him.

'Are you on remand?'

'Yes,' he replied, in his unhurried, unflustered manner. 'I've been charged with murder.'

For some reason the nurses had failed to warn me. I stopped tapping my keys and sunk into the back of my chair, giving David my full attention. I sensed that he was keen to explain why he had committed such a dreadful crime, and that he wanted to talk about it, otherwise he would not have mentioned it.

'Do you want to tell me what happened?' I asked gently.

I wondered if this was how priests felt when they were taking confession.

He closed his eyes for a moment, reliving the memory.

'I didn't mean to do it. I didn't plan it. I was overcome with rage and just grabbed a knife and . . .' His voice became so quiet that it was hard to hear. 'I stabbed him, I stabbed my father.'

He stared into my eyes, expecting a reaction. He didn't get one. I wasn't fazed by what he had admitted, and I certainly didn't feel threatened by him. David had a gentleness. His eyes were kind. I wondered what drove a man like him to kill his own father.

'I'd had enough,' he continued, his voice quivering a little. 'He'd bullied and belittled me my whole life. It had been building for years. I just . . . before I knew it, I'd killed him.'

He took a breath, but despite such a confession, remained surprisingly calm. He didn't appear mentally unbalanced, simply relieved that the years of torment were over.

I smiled sympathetically. What more could I do?

I was certain that the calmness he was exuding meant that the reality of what he had done, and where he was, hadn't sunk in yet. There would likely be fallout further down the line, especially as he must have been facing a very long sentence for killing his father.

But for now it seemed as if he wanted to brush all of his

pain under the carpet and talk about his life. We chatted as if we were friends meeting in the pub. It felt quite bizarre.

He told me that he'd always worked closely with his father and that they'd run a very successful cash and carry warehouse in Calais called Eastenders, selling cheap alcohol and cigarettes, and his father was dubbed the 'king of the booze cruise'.

I'd been to their warehouse many years ago; David and I used to make an annual trip to stock up on wine and beer. It was slightly surreal to be sitting opposite the man we'd probably bought wine from all those years ago. He continued to tell me of how his father bullied, humiliated and controlled him, and of how he'd made him feel worthless and never good enough.

The saddest thing of all was to see how relieved David seemed to be. That being there in the Scrubs was better than the abuse he'd suffered for years.

Perhaps a lot of people could relate to a time in their life when their family, or a business partner, or a loved one, had pushed them to the brink. But few of us, I would think, have been driven to quite that sort of desperate, all-consuming need to make the aggressor stop. To finally bring the abuse to an end, whatever the cost.

My conversation with David came to an abrupt end. There was an eruption of shouting and clanging gates, as the officers hurried the last of the new prisoners to their cells.

Terry appeared at my door.

'Locking up time, Doc!'

'Two seconds,' I said, buying myself a moment to check one last time that David was going to be okay. It always alarmed me when people were unnaturally calm during their first time in the nick.

'If you need anything, the nurses will be here all night to help you,' I reassured him.

He nodded and thanked me. Slowly, he rose to his feet, then disappeared from my room in the same unhurried manner that he had arrived, dragging behind him the plastic bag which contained all he had left from his former life.

The chances of our seeing one another again were slim. But I was glad we had met, and I hoped that he'd find peace.

Terry popped his nose around my door again.

'Locking up time, Doc!' he said with a big grin and extra emphasis. 'You need to get moving.'

'Two minutes,' I said, bartering for extra time. Before I logged out of my computer there was something I quickly needed to check.

I shook my head in disbelief. 'Wow!'

I had been right about Abdi being very seriously ill, but was surprised to find out that he was suffering from TB meningitis. Pulmonary TB – when tuberculosis affects the lungs – was not uncommon in the Scrubs, but never, in over thirty years of medicine, had I seen a case of TB meningitis – a much more serious, life-threating disease, that causes inflammation of the membranes around the brain and the spinal cord.

The hospital report stated that he was going to require a

lengthy course of treatment. He wouldn't be returning to the Scrubs; the treatment would outlast the rest of his sentence.

I would never know if he would make a full recovery, but at least my insistence to admit him to hospital had been correct.

'Come on, Doc!' Terry had returned to collect me, again.

I unhooked my jacket from the back of the chair, threading my weary arms through the sleeves. I hoisted my bag over my shoulder and gave Terry the nod to lead the way. We were clocking off together, so it was nice to have a bit of company as I walked to my car.

*

I stopped at the service station for a snack. My stomach had been talking to me in low growls for hours. For some reason the air conditioning was on full blast. I buttoned my jacket and hugged myself to keep warm as I waited in the queue.

To my right were rows of chocolate bars and sweets, tempting me to add them to my late-night munchies. Above were the CCTV monitors, flashing images of the pumps on the forecourt.

The man in front of me ordered a pack of Marlboro Lights and a scratch card. We all looked liked zombies, walking around so late at night in the unforgiving strip lighting.

I paid for my sandwich and made my way back through the shop to my car, keen to get back on the road and home.

By the door there were piles of the previous day's

newspapers, bundled together with string, soon to be turned into pulp. Staring up at me, was David West's face.

Above it read the headline – 'Son of flamboyant self-styled "Lord" David West is charged with murder after "stabbing to death" the nightclub owner at his Mayfair home.'

I hadn't realised that David's father had named his son after himself. In smaller print, the newspaper detailed how David West senior, 70, had died of a single knife wound at his £2.5million home.

I considered asking the cashier if he could cut me free a copy, but I thought better of it. I didn't need to know any more than David had told me himself. I wasn't interested in reading about the sordid details.

Instead, I carried on walking, past the pile of papers, through the glass doors and into the night.

Chapter Twenty

'The black or the blue?' I asked David, waving a trouser suit in either hand.

Squinting at me, my husband croaked, 'They look identical to me.'

'The black one then,' I decided, slipping the other hanger back into my wardrobe.

He rolled over while I carried on getting dressed. A flutter of nerves danced through my stomach. I sprayed a halo of perfume around my body and crept over to David, who had fallen fast asleep again. I kissed his cheek and he stirred. 'Good luck, you'll be fine.'

I hoped I would be. It should just have been a formality that I needed to get through, but I was so nervous. David's words, as always, had a calming effect on me.

I listened to Classic FM all the way into London, the sound of the beautiful music soothing my soul.

Despite setting off early to beat the rush-hour traffic, it was really difficult to find a parking space. I circled several times before I found one, and with every lap my anxiety cranked up a notch. I couldn't be late.

I stepped out into the bright sunshine, ironing the creases on my trousers with my hand, and looked up.

But that morning's view wasn't the towering walls of HMP Wormwood Scrubs. I was in a tree-lined street of semi-detached houses, in the affluent area of Fulham, West London.

In twenty minutes I was due to give evidence at the Coroner's Court. Another wave of anxiety rolled through me. I had to get a move on; I'd parked miles away.

I was soon out of breath, and my heart was pounding as I looked left and right along the busy main road.

'Come on, come on,' I hissed at the traffic lights, impatient to cross.

I glanced at my watch again. I hated being late.

I saw a clearing in the traffic and took my chances.

I sprinted across the road, but the heel of my shoe caught in my trousers and I tripped up, falling flat onto the hard concrete.

I looked up and, to my horror, a motorcycle was zipping around the corner. I braced myself for impact, but the roaring of the engine turned to a purr as it pulled over beside me.

'Are you okay?' the man on the bike asked, flicking up his visor as he dismounted to help me onto my feet.

'Yes, I'm fine, thank you' I said, feeling deeply embarrassed. My knees and hands were throbbing as I hobbled to the side of the road.

I thanked the man for being so kind and continued on my way, trying to salvage what was left of my dignity by straightening my jacket and dusting off my trousers. The shock of the fall had left me feeling even more shaky and anxious. Coupled with the adrenaline from running late, I was a total bag of nerves. I checked my hands for cuts and noticed they were trembling.

'Deep breath,' I said to myself as I walked towards the entrance of West London Coroner's Court.

It was an ugly red-brick building, which seemed out of place located in the middle of a quiet residential area of pretty houses.

It reminded me of the swimming baths I used to go to when I was little. An equally flustered-looking man was having a last few puffs on his cigarette on the steps. I wondered if he was a member of the deceased's family. I gave him a nod and then pushed my way through the big black doors that led inside.

The whitewashed corridor was a hive of activity. Solicitors and barristers were milling around. Everyone was looking very serious and official, carrying files of paperwork. There was a small group of smartly dressed people hovering by the door to court one, speaking in hushed tones. I wasn't sure who they were. Perhaps family. Or worse, journalists.

I searched the crowd for a friendly face, but she found me first.

'Amanda!' My boss, Karen, waved.

'It's been delayed by fifteen minutes.' She noticed my flustered state. 'You look like you could do with a coffee, are you okay?'

'Yes, I'm fine,' I replied. 'I just took a bit of a tumble on the way here. I have been dreading today, and hardly slept all night fretting about it.'

'I'm sure there's nothing to worry about,' Karen reassured me.

I was required to give evidence in court following the death of a man in Wormwood Scrubs about eighteen months previously. He had died in the FNC, and I was the only doctor who had seen him.

Suddenly the court door opened – our cue to go in.

'It won't take long,' Karen said as we queued to enter.

'I certainly hope not,' I said. 'I feel so anxious I can hardly think straight.'

There had been nothing remarkable about Daniel Craven's behaviour when he had walked into Reception that night, dragging his big bag of belongings.

He was polite and friendly, but the thing I most remembered about him was that, despite looking very dishevelled, he was wearing a smart designer jacket. Somehow the two just didn't seem to marry up.

It wasn't Daniel's first time in prison. One of the officers, Bill, recognised him. The two of them chatted away as if they were old mates, while I finished writing up my notes. I joined in the end of the conversation, remarking to Bill about the lovely jacket Daniel was wearing, which seemed to please him, as a big smile spread across his face and he proudly announced that he had bought it in a charity shop the previous week.

He told me he didn't have any illnesses that he knew of, he wasn't a drug user, and he wasn't on any medication. It was a little challenging at times to get a straight answer out of him, as he tended to go off on a tangent and talk about random things, but he certainly wasn't acting in an unusual way, and gave no cause for concern.

So you can imagine my surprise when at 9 a.m. the next morning, just as I was about to head off to the Seg to do the rounds, I heard alarm bells screeching and officers stampeding along the corridors shouting 'Code Blue!'

Daniel's dead body had been discovered, curled up around the lavatory in his cell.

Reports from staff working in the First Night Centre stated that he had grown increasingly agitated as the evening had worn on, so much so that they suspected he may have been smoking spice.

But the toxicology report didn't find a trace of any drug in his system. I wondered whether he may have had a stroke, a fit, a heart attack, but it was none of those either. It took months for the autopsy report to come back and, when it did, it stated that no cause of death had been identified.

It was a total mystery, and the first time in all my years since qualifying in medicine that I had encountered a death in which the cause could not to be identified.

*

I sat on the wooden bench, my legs crossed, my hands planted on my knees, waiting for my name to be called. The room was high-ceilinged, wood-panelled and brightly lit. In front of me was the witness box where all the people involved in the inquiry would take it in turns to give their accounts of what had happened that night.

Opposite the witness box was the jury, and to the left were rows of seats for the deceased's family and friends. Behind them were seats for members of the public.

The legal teams sat in the front two rows. Beyond the witness box, on a raised platform, was the coroner's desk.

Everyone stood up when he walked in. He was a short, bespectacled man, his black hair salted with grey. His face was crumpled, his expression frosty. His job was to investigate the circumstances surrounding the death, and to ensure there was no negligence or foul play. To make sure that if any fault was found, that everyone would learn from it. He would make recommendations after hearing the case, possibly suggesting certain prison procedures should change, to try to avoid another tragedy.

I glanced across to the bench where the family would sit, but it was empty and my heart sank.

I wondered if Daniel, like many of the prisoners I met, didn't have any family, or had no one who cared enough to come to his inquest, and the thought made me feel so sad.

'Doctor Brown.' My name echoed off the high ceiling.

I slowly rose to my feet, clutching my notes in my right hand, and made my way to the box. I looked to Karen and she gave me an encouraging smile. My heart was racing and my hands were shaking. My mouth was so dry I was worried I wouldn't be able to speak.

It started well. I was questioned by the barrister representing the Scrubs. He was there to defend me, not to try to trip me up. I told the court the little I knew about Daniel Craven.

'There really isn't anything more I can add,' I eventually concluded.

'Thank you, Doctor Brown,' the lawyer said, nodding to the coroner that he had finished his questions.

The lawyer for the Crown Prosecution Service then stood up. She was young, mid-thirties and immaculately dressed. Her blonde hair was tied back into a tight chignon bun. She stared back at me with cold, steely eyes.

Clearing her throat, she said, 'Doctor Brown, could you please tell us again your impressions of Mr Craven on the night you saw him.'

I glanced down at the notes, balancing on the small wooden ledge inside the witness box.

'Of course,' I replied politely, although inside I was feeling increasingly frustrated that I had to keep running through a story that had very little to it. As far as I was concerned, I felt the focus should have been on the rest of the evening, on those hours Daniel was in the First Night Centre, reportedly growing increasingly agitated.

I hadn't fully understood the meaning of the word cross-examined until then. Ninety minutes later I was still in the witness box, repeatedly going over every minute detail of those fifteen minutes I had spent with him in Reception.

In the end it all became a bit of blur. I felt under attack. I felt criticised. More than anything else I felt angry that I was made to feel guilty, as if I had done something wrong, in front of a whole room full of people. There was only one question that I remember clearly, one that cut deep.

The coroner interrupted the CPS lawyer to ask me a question himself. Peering over his glasses, the frosty-faced man said, 'Why would you have reason to go back into the notes, Doctor Brown?'

He was referring to the fact that I had logged into Daniel's medical records after I had finished seeing him. It was something I nearly always did after I had seen someone, to make sure I had typed the notes up correctly, that the sentences made sense and that there were no spelling mistakes. There was often a lot of pressure on the doctors, from the officers, to get the prisoners processed as quickly as possible, and so I usually checked the notes to make sure that I hadn't made any errors in my rush.

But I was taken aback by the coroner's line of questioning. I felt as if he was implying that I had tried to cover something up. Maybe I was taking it too personally, and he just needed to understand my reasons for rechecking the notes, but with the tension I was feeling I was struggling to think clearly.

A deathly silence hung in the air, awaiting my answer. I froze. The words caught in my throat and I couldn't speak.

With every second that ticked by I felt increasingly self-conscious, and as if everyone in the room was thinking that I had done something wrong.

I felt so hurt, as I care passionately about doing the right thing, but at that moment I felt unworthy and useless.

Thoughts tumbled through my head, but I still couldn't speak. I knew in my heart that that there was nothing I could have done differently that night that would have made a difference.

I felt as if I was going to pass out. Finally, I managed to answer his question, and I held myself together until the nightmare was over and there were no more questions.

I clung on to my composure as I left the witness box. But with every step my legs turned more to jelly.

Karen gestured that she would meet me outside the courtroom. I followed her in silence, feeling everyone's eyes trailing after me, judging me. Although in reality they were probably fixed on the next witness being sworn in.

I let out a little gasp of relief as soon as I reached the noisy corridor. I could breathe again.

'Well done,' Karen said, softly. 'You did so well.'

I smiled weakly and suddenly it hit me how utterly drained I felt.

Karen gave me a hug and my composure cracked. I wrapped my arms around her and sobbed.

'I can't do this any more,' I whispered, when I could eventually speak.

She stroked my back soothingly. 'It's okay, it's done, it's over.'

But the experience wasn't over for me. I couldn't just shrug it off as I had with so many of the prison dramas. It had knocked my confidence. But most of all, it had rocked that deep insecurity of mine to the core, and I had never felt so undervalued and useless in my life.

Chapter Twenty-One

In all my previous thirty years of practising medicine, before working in prisons, I had never had to attend a Coroner's Court. But in the seven years I had been at the Scrubs, I had been required to attend on four occasions.

Somehow, rather than becoming less daunting, each time I attended I found it more and more stressful.

The shine had been taken off the Scrubs.

I dreaded having to attend another Coroner's Court, and became almost paranoid about writing even more meticulous notes on everybody that I saw.

The fear of missing something was almost crippling.

I worried that someone was going to find fault with me. I'd been told to walk with confidence when in prison. Now I felt like I was walking on eggshells all the time.

The situation became worse not long after the court case, as a vicious batch of spice was doing the rounds.

The effects were extreme, and the men that used it either became zombie-like or wild and very aggressive. Some were having fits and losing consciousness.

I was terrified for the men's safety, and I feared that

sooner or later someone might die as a result of smoking spice.

It was so bad that alarm bells were going off everywhere, and I spent my time going from one wing to another, seeing prisoners who were either recovering from the effects of it, or who were having to be restrained by officers.

As doctors we were helpless to do anything. Sometimes we would send them to hospital, only for the doctors there to send them straight back to prison, saying they couldn't help; the drug needed to work its way out of their system.

The fear of further deaths took away the fun from a job I had once loved.

The final straw came one afternoon when I was called to C Wing for an emergency.

The nurses had helped one of the prisoners into the consultation room, after he had collapsed on the landing. They managed to get him onto the examination couch so that he could lie down.

He was skinny and pale, his face covered in blemishes with a nasty weeping cold sore on his bottom lip. He looked undernourished and as if he hadn't slept for weeks.

Sylvie was already by his side, waiting to fill me in on what had happened.

'Thank God you're here,' she said. 'Today has been a nightmare. It's one thing after another. What's happening to this place?' She shook her head, sagging with exhaustion.

'We found Alex having a fit on the landing. His notes are on the screen for you.' As I scanned the records, I could see Alex wasn't a stranger to prison. He'd been in and out since he was 15 years of age, and had some complex medical issues.

I initially suspected he might have suffered an epileptic fit, but he had no previous history of epilepsy.

'I think he's been on the old . . .' Sylvie rolled her eyes to the ceiling, in frustration. I instinctively knew she was referring to spice.

'I'll never use it again, Doc,' he murmured, then started retching violently. 'I feel so sick.'

He clutched his stomach, a thick string of saliva trailing between his mouth and the couch.

His hair was bright ginger. His face was so white he looked like a corpse. Even his lips were drained of colour.

In the ruthless world of prison drug dealing, it was usually the most vulnerable who suffered. Dealers sometimes wanted to test their merchandise, to see what effects it would have. They would often offer a 'free' sample to those with learning difficulties, or other vulnerabilities. Or they would simply force them to take the drug, to see what happened.

I wondered if the young man had been cherry-picked to be a guinea pig.

With anxiety in his voice, he explained. 'I couldn't sleep one night. Someone offered me a joint and it got me to sleep. The next night I thought it was a good idea, and that's how I got hooked.'

He stared at me with desperate eyes, looking for sympathy. 'When you can't sleep it's like you're doing double time.'

I'd heard the term 'double time' on many occasions over the years, usually when the prisoners were desperately hoping that I would be able to prescribe them sleeping pills. I could imagine it must have been like having a double sentence, if the nights lasted as long as the days. Probably even more painful for those in the Seg.

'When I do drugs, I don't feel nothing. I don't see nothing. That's why I use; it makes me forget I'm here. It blocks everything out. I shut my eyes. I feel calm and relaxed. I can't even move. It takes over, and the time flies, it absolutely flies,' Alex said, before he started retching again. 'But I've never used spice before, and I'm never going to use it again. Never!'

There was nothing I could do for him. I didn't know how the drug had reacted, and the last thing I wanted to do was give him another drug that could make things worse. He just had to let it work itself out of his system.

I appreciated his honesty in admitting that he had used illicit drugs, as he knew that he could be punished for it. By telling me the truth he had spared me a lot of time considering alternative causes for his collapse, and possibly from sending him to hospital for further investigation and monitoring.

That day I realised that the frighteningly rapid rise of the use of spice throughout the prison was out of control, and that I could no longer continue to work there.

My time was up.

*

I had loved working in the Scrubs. I loved the banter, the noise, the excitement. I loved belonging somewhere. I loved the fact that the officers and a lot of the prisoners knew me. I was such a familiar sight around the prison that I felt like part of the fixtures and fittings. It was a really hard decision to make, but one that I knew was right. After seven years in the notorious Victorian prison, I decided it was time to leave.

I don't like big goodbyes because I get very emotional. So I didn't let many people know I was going. Only my very closest friends at the Scrubs knew that the August bank holiday of 2016 was going to be my last day there.

As always, David was fully supportive of my leaving, and of my decision to not give up working behind bars. Instead I had decided to face my biggest fear of all – working in a women's prison.

Many officers and medical staff had warned me not to do so, saying that female prisoners could be much more challenging, with a very high rate of self-harm. Governor Frake had given me some hard truths, having worked in the infamous Holloway for sixteen years. She said she much preferred dealing with men, and that I'd have my work cut out for me. But it was time to try something new.

So I signed up for some shifts in HMP Bronzefield, a closed female prison in Ashford. It is now the largest high-security female prison in Europe, since the closure of HMP Holloway.

Female prisons are not categorised in the same way as male prisons, and are referred to instead as either Closed or Open.

Opened in 2004, the modern building is a huge contrast to the Scrubs. The prison is divided into four house blocks, each housing up to 135 women. It also has a twelve-bed Mother and Baby Unit, accommodating children up to eighteen months old. Unlike in the Scrubs, the Number One Governor is referred to as the Director, the prisoners as residents, and the Seg as Separation and Care.

*

As I took my last steps on my final shift in the Scrubs I felt incredibly sad. It was the end of an era, but I had made my decision and was looking forward to the next chapter in my life.

I was walking down the grated metal steps to the ground floor of B Wing, my bag slung over my shoulder, my feet weary from another long day, when all of a sudden the place exploded with bangs and shouts from every direction. It sounded like a riot had broken out.

'You fucking blinder!' from my right.

'Get in!' from my left.

'Eeeeengland!' from above.

It was the explosive sound that I had become so used to whenever there was a football match on TV. When a goal was scored the place erupted and the noise was deafening. It always made me smile. In that moment, there were a lot of happy people in the Scrubs.

As I approached the exit gates, one of the prison officers was grinning.

'England just scored!' he said. 'Worst thing about being on duty is I don't get to watch the game.'

'Bad luck,' I replied as I reached for my keys, but kindly he stepped forward.

'Here, let me.' The keys rattling in that old lock. It would be the last time I heard it.

'Night, Doc,' he said. 'Safe journey home.'

I smiled back, but the smile didn't reach inside. 'Goodnight.'

I disappeared from the prison. Whether I had left a mark I didn't know. But I hoped I had, in my own small way, helped some of those men.

I was going to miss it. All of it.

PART THREE

HMP Bronzefield
2016–present

Chapter Twenty-Two

It was New Year's Day and, as I unlocked the final set of iron doors and gates that led to the Healthcare Centre, I had an unusual glimmer of hope.

The hope that maybe, just maybe, some of the women that I had seen returning to prison time and time again might not be coming back. That some may manage to break the vicious circle of drugs, crime and homelessness that so many had been stuck in for years.

My morning clinic was fully booked but my upbeat mood was soon squashed when I saw Jane's name on my list.

I had become very fond of Jane and felt deeply sorry for her.

She was 21 years of age, tall, attractive, highly intelligent and articulate. Sadly, she had extremely complex mental-health issues and an extensive and varied history of self-harm, which included cutting her arms, burning herself with boiling water and swallowing cutlery and pens.

In her young life she had swallowed so many foreign bodies that she had undergone twenty gastroscopies to retrieve them. On her last admission she was told that surgery was becoming increasingly hazardous, and that she somehow had to try to stop doing it. As soon as she came into my room, with her flat expression and empty stare, I knew she had self-harmed again. This time she had swallowed a plastic knife and fork. She said very little, but I had grown to understand her and didn't need to ask her too much, which she appreciated. *What a sad and tragic life,* I thought, as I made arrangements for her to be admitted to hospital again.

After lunch I went to Reception to see the new arrivals from court and was greeted by Helen.

'Happy New Year, Doc!' she said with a cheery smile. She was soon to be released after serving two years for fraud, and was one of the prisoners who worked in Reception, earning from £2.40 to £3.20 per day depending on the job. Helen's job was dispensing the 'welcome packs' for the newcomers. Each pack contained: a plastic knife, fork, plate and mug; unbranded shampoo, toothpaste, toothbrush, soap, hair conditioner and hairbrush; six new pairs of knickers, six pairs of socks, two T-shirts, two tracksuits, two sweatshirts and a nightie; and a pack of tea and sugar. The prisoner's worldly possessions could all be contained in one white fishnet sack.

I had about ten minutes to get myself set up in the small windowless consultation room, before starting to see the stream of new prisoners who had arrived from court. Many of them were likely to be withdrawing from drugs and alcohol.

I started along the familiar corridor, harshly lit by strip lights, my shoes squeaking against the mottled blue lino flooring. The tired white walls, smudged with black scuff marks. The slightly nauseating blend of microwaved meals and instant coffee wafted my way. The meals were offered to new arrivals because they would most likely get to the the house block too late to get a meal from the servery.

To my left there was a notice board with picture illustrations of the prisoner payment system.

Further down on the right was the room in which the new residents were waiting to be seen, and to my left was what looked like a shop counter where their possessions were checked and stored. Hajon and Jenny, two lovely officers, smiled and greeted me with a cheery 'Hi, Doc.'

'Busy today?' I asked them. I was hoping that there would not be too many new arrivals on New Year's Day.

'It's not looking too bad, Doc,' Hajon replied. 'Only ten due in.'

On a Bank Holiday only the magistrates' courts, not the Crown Courts, were open. On a normal day up to thirty new residents could arrive, so ten was an easy number to deal with.

As I walked past the glass window of the waiting room, another voice cut across the din with a sense of urgency and a thick Essex accent.

''Ello, Doctor Brown . . .'

The voice was so familiar I didn't need to see her to know who it belonged to. My heart sank.

It had only been five days since I had last seen Paula, to sign off her prescription on release from prison. Five days since she'd walked free. When we last met, she had been wearing make-up, her thick chestnut hair was washed and braided neatly into a plait, her eyes bright and full of hope. She was going to make it this time on the outside, she had said.

She couldn't have looked more different now, slumped in her uniform tracksuit. Her eyes were puffy and red, her long hair dirty and bedraggled, half covering her face. I couldn't see her arms but I suspected they'd have new needle marks.

Paula had already been screened by the nurse in Reception, so was the first to be seen. I called her in.

'Good to see you, Doc,' she said through her tears.

I looked at her forehead and was pleased to see that she hadn't cut herself this time, but I knew that she might if I didn't give her the correct medication quickly. Paula usually self-harmed by cutting her forehead. The compulsion would descend whenever she was frustrated and overwhelmed by emotions, and, of course whenever she was feeling ill when withdrawing from drugs and alcohol.

She'd left on a 50ml methadone script, but I guessed she probably hadn't been to a chemist to collect it, either because she couldn't be bothered or, more likely, because she had started using heroin again as she was still homeless.

So many of the women that I treated for drug and alcohol addiction in prison were homeless, and early on I realised that homelessness was very often the underlying cause of the seemingly never-ending circle of drugs, crime and prison. One lady once told me that if she was homeless after being released from prison, she would almost certainly get back on drugs as the only shelter she would find would be in a crack house, and to get into a crack house she had to have drugs to give the person running the crack house and to use herself while in there.

Many had also told me that they wanted to get back into prison so that they could sleep in a bed.

Paula had an extensive medical history. By the age of 38 she had been addicted to alcohol, cocaine and heroin for over twenty years. She was diagnosed with hepatitis C in 2010, but had never had treatment, mainly due to her chaotic lifestyle.

She had been in and out of prison from the age of 18. The longest sentence she'd received was six years at the age of 21, of which she served four years ten months. Most of her crimes had been theft to fund her drug habit. Thieving from shops, supermarkets – grabbing anything she could get her hands on in order to survive, and to trade for crack or heroin.

Unlike most of the women I met, she had a good child-hood and had attended an all-girls grammar school. She had always felt secure, but then her life went completely off the rails at the age of 15, when her father left home for another woman. This shock was the catalyst for her decline.

She started to hang around with the wrong crowd, an older group of so-called friends, who introduced her to drugs. She started off using cannabis but soon was smoking and then injecting heroin and crack, and so the dependency began.

She had broken down in tears when she recounted the horror of how she had been injected with drugs and then sexually abused, and then had fallen into despair when the drugs wore off and the reality of what had happened sunk in.

'They left me for dead in a park,' she sobbed, as she told me how she'd woken on a freezing cold day to find the buttons on her shirt had been torn off. Her bra was twisted, exposing her breasts to everyone who passed by.

'I was falling in and out of consciousness, but I could feel the pain inside me from where they had raped me. It was burning, but I couldn't move.'

She had been helped by a random passer-by, who had taken her to hospital, but no amount of medication could heal the emotional wounds inflicted on her. Paula's self-worth evaporated and her life had spiralled out of control.

'My real demon is crack, Doc.'

She told me how she had spent as much as £200 a day on the crystal form of cocaine. 'It blocks out the memories. It takes away the pain. You understand, don't you, Doc?'

Sadly, I understood that kind of self-destructive behaviour all too well, as I had heard it from so many women.

Paula was a warm, intelligent, articulate woman, with a lovely sense of humour, and on the many times I saw her she talked of wanting to sort her life out. She genuinely wanted to change her life, but she kept falling into her old ways on release as that was the only life she knew.

I'd followed her through her highs and her lows, and grown to really like her. I wanted to see her get back on her feet, and every time she disappeared from my room, I was willing her to find the strength to change.

I braced myself for the latest chapter in her tragic story.

She looked exhausted. Strip lighting doesn't flatter anyone but she looked particularly careworn, the pronounced lines under her eyes adding at least ten years to her age.

'Doc, I don't know how to cope when I get out of here any more.'

Paula broke down again in tears, and I looked around the room for a box of tissues. To my frustration there wasn't one. So I ripped a clean piece of blue paper towel from the examination couch and handed her a big wodge of it.

'Here you go, lovely,' I said.

She blew her nose loudly, then managed to squeeze out a smile. I put my arm around her shoulders to try to comfort her.

I needed to go through the routine questions on the computer template . . . why was she in prison? Sentenced or remand? If sentenced, how long for, etc. This was the ninth time I had seen Paula in Reception in the past eighteen months, and I could fill out almost every box without even asking her for the details.

Paula buried her head into her hands as she repeated:

'I don't know how to survive. I just don't know how to do it.'

It was clear that Paula wanted to turn her life around, but couldn't see a way out. She was looking to me for answers, but I had none. I had learnt over the years that often the best and most helpful thing I could do was listen, and let people pour their problems out to me.

'So what have you done this time?' I asked gently.

Paula's eyes dropped to the floor. I could tell she felt ashamed as she withdrew into the back of the hard brown plastic chair. She tugged at one of her knotted strands of hair as she began to tell me how things had fallen apart after leaving the prison.

'I planned to stay with my mum but that didn't work out, so I was back on the streets and it was freezing. I was sleeping in a bin store in Ashford, not far from the prison.'

It was terrible to think of her, two days after Christmas, alone and homeless. She'd become so institutionalised that she felt safer near the prison than in her own home town.

As I had suspected, Paula hadn't made it to a pharmacy to stay on methadone, and had gone back on heroin. She was back in prison for nicking booze and food from a local supermarket.

'I thought I was having a nervous breakdown because I was imagining people following me, and then they weren't there. I'm paranoid. Do you think I'm paranoid?' she rattled on, breathlessly.

She had no history of psychosis in her notes, but I'd seen before the erratic behaviour that accompanied withdrawal from drugs and alcohol. Paranoia was common enough.

Her arms bore the scars of deep knife wounds, where she had cut herself out of frustration. Her skin was criss-crossed with lacerations. The wounds on her forehead were more superficial than on her arms, but sadly much more visible – a tattoo to her misery.

Almost certainly, if she had not fallen out with her mum, and had somewhere to live, she would have stood a chance to get off drugs and stay out of prison. But, as she had confided in me some while ago, although she adored her mother she found it hard to spend time with her, because of her mum's partner.

'He tried it on with me when my mum was out at the shops. I told him to take his hands off me, that he was a dirty bastard for wanting me when he's with my mum! He lost his temper and smacked me across the face. I fell and whacked my head on the corner of the couch. He grabbed a fistful of my hair and tried to push my head down as he climbed on my back but I wasn't going to let him get me. I kicked him and I bit into his arm, and I managed to free myself and run for the door.'

It was yet another story of a man taking advantage of her vulnerability. I sensed this encounter had hurt her more than some of the other abuse she had suffered – probably because she had been thrust into a situation that could potentially cause problems to her already fractured relationship with her mother.

Paula had narrowly avoided being raped, but she couldn't bring herself to tell her mum.

'She wouldn't believe me anyway, Doc – she'll do anything to keep him.'

But it was not just the boyfriend that made Paula wary of visiting her mum. A big part of what was keeping Paula from getting help was shame. She didn't want her mum to see what a mess she was in, physically and mentally. She felt ashamed of the woman she had become, so she hid herself amongst the people who didn't care about her, who fed her addictions.

I didn't go into too much depth about her crime this time around. Usually it was the same old thing with Paula – stealing alcohol. She drunk heavily to numb the pain of her past. She stole food because she was starving.

She'd spent two nights in police custody, before appearing in front of the magistrates' court, where they were familiar with her previous history and sentenced her to another six weeks in prison.

I could tell she was embarrassed to be back in custody after insisting it was going to be different this time. Of course, she'd believed it would.

Her eyes were still glued to the floor as I asked her questions about something she refused to address – her hepatitis C.

She found it hard to look at me, because she knew she needed treatment and felt guilty that she was doing nothing to help herself.

People can contract hep C if they share needles, so sadly it is not an uncommon problem with drug users. Fortunately,

Paula's liver was still functioning normally, as her bloods had been checked when she was last in prison and no abnormality was detected. Nor was she displaying any signs of liver failure, and although a small percentage of people with hep C recover with no treatment, she was scared that if she didn't get help sooner or later it might kill her. Sadly, rather than tackling the problem, she stuck her head in the sand and did nothing about it.

Instead she continued to drink very heavily when she wasn't in prison, to try to keep warm and to block out her fears, thoughts and memories – which of course was terrible for her liver, so it was remarkable that it was still functioning normally.

The only way for Paula to get treatment would be by being in one place for a few months, but she was never either in or out of prison for long enough to get help. Six weeks being locked up behind bars might feel like a lifetime for some, but it was not enough time for me to help Paula get treatment. By the end of her sentence in Bronzefield, the best I could hope for was to have her stable on methadone. Only she could decide when to change her life.

I prescribed all her medication, and as she got up to leave she gave me a big, tearful hug.

'God bless ya, Doc,' she said.

Relief washed across her face as she turned to me and said, 'I feel at home here.'

I realised the drugs weren't her only addiction. She had become dependent on the safety that prison gave her. It was almost unbearably sad.

Chapter Twenty-Three

To begin with, my job in Bronzefield was based in the Healthcare department, running GP clinics and seeing new arrivals in Reception. Very rarely was I called to attend emergencies on the house blocks. In general those were dealt with by the nurses.

The shifts were 9.30 a.m. to 4.30 p.m. in the week days (although I never completed the work in this time), or until 9 p.m. if the shift included a Reception session in the evening. The work was varied, exhausting, and often emotionally draining, but without doubt it was very rewarding.

There were five other doctors sharing the work, and I worked on average three days a week.

The first job of the day was to see the residents in Separation and Care, or those located in Healthcare, the rounds for each taking place on alternate days. After that I would start the clinic and see a range of different problems, including anyone who had arrived in custody too late the night before to have been seen by a GP in Reception. Those withdrawing from drugs or alcohol would be seen by the on-call doctor after 9 p.m. for their essential medication to be prescribed, but a full medical history would be postponed until the following day.

In the afternoon there was another full clinic booked, with routine medical problems, path results to file and action, and prescriptions to be rewritten.

The days were full on, but I was delighted by how many of the women wanted to open up to me. I found their stories fascinating, often tragic, and sometimes almost too shocking to comprehend. I became a shoulder to cry on for many of them, and I didn't mind a bit. On the contrary I felt privileged to hear their stories and invariably humbled by them. At times we also shared some wonderful laughter, especially when they used expressions (often very rude!) that I had never heard before!

My fears of working in a female prison had been completely unfounded. I felt accepted by the women from the very first day I worked there, and flattered that they felt they could relate to me. One of the nicest things they might say when the consultation was over would be, 'Thank you for not judging me.'

Some were lonely and frightened, but many of the regulars seemed happy to chat and often shared a joke. I was also amazed by how many women told me that they felt safer in prison than outside.

One lady told me that she had been in a violent controlling relationship for the past seven years, and that her first night in prison was the first time she had felt safe in bed for seven years!

Another said that she felt more free in prison than outside, as she was free from the man who had controlled her for the past twelve years.

Horrible and shocking.

I soon realised that a high percentage of the women in prison were actually victims, and that was perhaps the most striking thing about female prisoners. Their stories of abuse, of being beaten, raped, and controlled both physically and mentally were deeply disturbing.

Before I started working there I was concerned that the women might have perceived me to be from a privileged background, and therefore assumed that I would not be able to understand their struggles. The fact that they chose to confide in me was wonderful.

The crimes they were being punished for committing were often a direct result of the abuse they'd suffered. I'd heard women explain how they'd killed their partner, after years of abuse, to protect themselves or safeguard their children. Countless women, like Paula, revealed how they were stuck in an endless cycle of drug addiction and crime which began after being abused. The memories of the abuse still haunted them, and they couldn't stop turning to drugs to numb the pain, to blot out time, to stamp out the memories. It was either that or self-harming. Or worse: trying to take their own lives, which a lot of the women had attempted to do at some point.

In April 2017 I was asked to run the Substance Misuse Clinic on House Block One. In a strange way I saw this as my final demon to face, as although I had the necessary qualifications to do it I genuinely did not want to.

This stemmed from the fact that, up until then, my only contact with substance misusers was in Reception, when they were usually feeling extremely unwell due to withdrawal symptoms.

Some of them managed to engage in a polite and coherent manner, but many were rude, demanding, angry, irritable, and just desperate to get medication to stop them feeling so dreadful. I understood and empathised but, honestly, didn't relish the idea of working with such angry and abusive prisoners.

To my astonishment I found that I enjoyed the work, and soon realised how lovely most of the women were when they were no longer feeling so ill from withdrawal. Their stories were awful and sad, but so touching and important to share. I began to understand more and more about the physical and emotional dependency they had on drugs.

A lovely lady called Andrea explained that using heroin was like being wrapped in a warm blanket that made her feel safe and protected.

'It's like eating Ready Brek.'

'Ready Brek? The breakfast cereal?' I asked.

'Yeah, you get that glow inside you. Like the advert, when they start glowing when they eat it. The feeling cocoons you, wraps its arms around you and makes everything feel safe. You can face your worst demons when you take heroin. It gives you strength. It's your best friend. It's your mum, your dad, it's every family member you've got . . . all rolled into one, there for you. That's what heroin feels like.

'All my problems, depression, anxieties, it locks them away in a box. You can stand back and look at them from afar and think they will take care of themselves, when you are on heroin.

'It gives you a false sense of life. Nothing is how it seems.'

She looked up at me through her hollowed eyes. 'It gives me the life I wish I had.'

Her words clung to the air, turning it heavy with tragedy.

What she hadn't said, her reason for needing to be cocooned by the drug, was the elephant in the room. Something awful had happened to Andrea. She was painfully thin and her eyes were haunted. As she sat opposite me it seemed as if she was drained of any emotion or feeling, as if she was exhausted by life.

I smiled at her. 'How long have you been using now?'

Andrea tucked a strand of her straggly blonde hair behind her ear. The roots were greasy, the ends were dry and split, and there wasn't much left of it.

'Twenty-five years,' she said, quietly. 'Although I've managed to stay clean for short periods of time.'

Some of the women who use said they felt ashamed of their habit and lifestyle, and were embarrassed to tell me for fear I might judge them.

'It's okay,' I reassured her.

She relaxed a little and then rolled up the sleeves of her jumper and showed me her arms, which were scarred and discoloured.

'I can't inject here any more, I've done it so much that all the veins in my arms and legs are too damaged.'

Fighting back the tears of shame, she slowly raised her finger and pointed to the tiny veins running underneath her eyes. 'So I inject here, it's the only place left.'

I was horrified.

'Oh, Andrea!'

She shook her head, trying to shake the tears away and swallowed hard, determined to retain her composure. Many of the women I'd seen in Bronzefield struggled to let down their guard. I suppose so many terrible things had happened to them when they did.

My job was to prescribe Andrea the correct dose of methadone to try to prevent the symptoms of heroin withdrawal which were making her feel so ill. But I also wanted to understand why she had started using drugs all those years ago. I asked her if there had been something that had triggered her to start using, or was it just the life she was leading at the time.

'I started when I was twenty-seven,' she said. 'After I was attacked with a claw hammer.'

I stared at her, shocked at what I was hearing.

'I was doing a talk on computer programming, and the company that had contracted me out had put me up in a hotel in London. When I was walking back to the hotel in the evening, two men tried to take my bag off me. But I wouldn't give it to them. Even though there was nothing much in there, I didn't want them to have it.'

Suddenly her voice started to crack.

'Have you got a tissue, Doctor Brown?'

I had come prepared with several packets. I rummaged in my bag and handed her one.

She dabbed the tears that had collected in the corners of her eyes. Struggling to get the words out, she said, 'I wished I'd just given it to them now.'

I nodded sympathetically. It was all I could do.

'When I wouldn't give in, one of them pulled out a claw hammer. It all happened so quickly, he pulled his arm back and smacked it down so hard on my head.'

I winced, imagining the horrifying scene.

Slowly, Andrea titled her head forward and pulled away some of her hair to reveal a marked indentation in the top of her skull.

'Oh my God,' I whispered.

'I felt so much pain, and then I didn't feel anything. Just the blood trickling down my face. I remember that being warm on my skin.

'I tried to get up but I couldn't move my legs. They wouldn't work. I thought the men had run off with my bag and left me there, but then I saw their shoes as they stood over me.

'I wanted to scream but I couldn't open my mouth, it just wouldn't open.'

Andrea's hands were shaking as she nervously wrapped the tissue around her fingers.

'One of the men wrenched me onto my feet, grabbed me

by both arms and dragged me along the street. I couldn't hold my head up and was barely conscious. I wanted to scream out but my mouth was clamped shut.'

Tears were streaming down Andrea's face, and they were welling in my eyes.

'I must have blanked out at that point because I don't remember how I got inside. When I opened my eyes I could see I was in a bedroom. It had a brown carpet and there were no sheets on the bed, just a stained mattress. One of the cupboard doors was open and I think there were clothes hanging in there. I tried to move my legs but they still weren't working. I tried to move my hands and that's when I realised, they had tied me to the radiator.

'They must have heard me move, as the two men appeared in the doorway, speaking in a foreign language. One of them started laughing. He had a beard and short hair and as he approached me I could smell him. There was an evil stench of booze as he breathed over me.

'He pulled at my jeans, tugging them down my legs, and I was helpless to do anything.' Andrea shook her head, sobbing, clutching the tissue tightly in a ball. 'I couldn't do anything to stop him.

'That blow to the head had paralysed part of my body. I could see it all happening to me but I couldn't scream, I couldn't move, I just had to let it happen.

'He unbuckled his belt and unzipped his jeans and I knew what was coming. I could still close my eyes so that's what I did. I shut them tightly and prayed it would be over soon.'

Tears were streaming down Andrea's cheeks and mine.

'For three days they kept me there, raping me.'

Her head collapsed into her hands as she sobbed and sobbed.

I felt physically sick hearing her story. I don't think I had ever heard anything quite so shocking. Whatever the reason Andrea was in prison, it took nothing away from the horror of what she had suffered.

I handed her my whole pack of tissues.

'Thank you.' She sniffed, wiping her tear-stained face.

For a moment we sat in silence – Andrea calming her emotions, me digesting the horror of what she had described.

When she finally spoke, she told me how, when the men were finished abusing her, they dumped her in a side street, next to some bags of rubbish. She woke up in hospital in excruciating pain.

'The surgeons had to take part of my skull away. I had to undergo major surgery. I was paralysed down one side of my body, and I was in hospital for months and had to learn to walk and talk again.'

'I can't get my head around this,' I said. 'Did they catch the men?'

'No, the police never found them, even though there was CCTV on the street. There had even been some witnesses.'

I shook my head in despair.

Andrea looked at me directly in the eye. 'I guess I'm lucky to be alive. They could have killed me.' And then she whispered, 'Some days, I wish they had.'

It was an awful thing to hear, but I understood. Andrea didn't need to explain to me why she had turned to drugs – to numb the physical and emotional scars.

'How long are you in here for?' I asked.

'I've been sentenced for eighteen months,' she said.

'Did you commit the crime to get money for drugs?'

She nodded, sheepishly.

'When was the last time you were in prison?'

'Fifteen years ago, I spent six months in Holloway.'

'You did well to stay out of prison for so long.'

'Yeah, I've tried. I've had jobs.' She sighed deeply. 'But I always end up going back on heroin, and then I lose them.

'The worst thing is the sleep. I still find it hard to sleep, as I still have flashbacks. And when I can't sleep everything seems worse and I end up back on the gear just to take me away from it all.

'I hate asking people for money, so I ended up doing lunch and dinner dates with people I met on the internet as an escort.

'I could earn £110 an hour,' she said, ashamedly.

'For sex?'

'Mostly it wasn't actual sex, that only happened once. But it was better than being in trouble with the police.'

Many of the women had told me that they had turned to prostitution to survive. One poor dishevelled soul had once said that she had been a prostitute for years, and matter-of-factly stated, 'I'm a machine. I don't feel anything any more.'

One had even told me that her mother had sent her out

for prostitution at the age of 14, to bring in money for the family; another that she had grown up in a brothel as her mum was a prostitute.

It explained how Andrea had managed to stay out of prison for so long, despite not holding down a job.

'But I had a big habit and I wasn't getting enough money, so I turned to crime again.'

Andrea had been in prison for two weeks and the 30ml of methadone was not holding her. She still felt sick, achey, had hot and cold sweats, diarrhoea and abdominal cramps.

'I don't really want to be on methadone,' she said. 'I wish I could go cold turkey as I know I've just swapped one habit for another, but I feel so dreadful. I think the only way to do it is to increase my meth and then try a slow detox when I feel stable.'

I had heard such a plan many times, and had realised early on when I started working with substance misusers that they all had their own ways of dealing with dependency. Some told me they could never imagine a life off drugs, others said that they were tired of it and wanted their lives back. I learned too that only *they* could decide when they were ready to stop using.

Very often their sentence was far too short to allow them to detox, and often the dose of methadone had to be increased – what's known as 'titrated up' – to a suitable dose to keep them safe from possible overdose after release.

I agreed to titrate the dose up and arranged to review her in three weeks' time.

She smiled weakly. 'Okay, Doc.'

Methadone is a green liquid which looks a bit like Fairy Liquid and I am told has a very unpleasant taste. Prisoners are given their methadone by the nurses at around 9 a.m., but if the dose is not sufficient it won't hold them through the full twenty-four hours, which is what was happening to Andrea.

In the past, all prisoners were expected to detox from methadone if they were due to remain in custody for more than three months, but this is no longer the case.

'Thanks, Doc.'

As Andrea got out of the chair, the tissue she'd been clutching so tightly fell to the floor. She bent over to pick it up, giving me a second glimpse of the dent in her head.

'Thank you again,' she said, her painfully thin body disappearing out of the door.

I had eighteen months to get her back on her feet. With Andrea, I had something to work with, unlike many of the other women who flitted in and out of the prison.

I couldn't help questioning though: was prison the right place for Andrea? For Paula? For all these women who were committing petty crimes to feed their drug habits? If only there could be a better support system for them when they left prison, perhaps they wouldn't need to turn to drugs again.

I was seeing the world from both sides of the prison walls, with new eyes.

Chapter Twenty-Four

Suzanne was putting me in a very difficult position.

'I can't cope without it, Doc, please, you have to give it to me,' she begged.

I had been warned that the drugs wing in a women's prison could be the hardest place of all to work, as so many of the women were emotionally unstable, as well as struggling with addiction. They would go to any lengths to get the drugs they had become addicted to. I realised how true this was, as they would so often tug at my heartstrings in a desperate bid to coerce me into prescribing what they wanted.

Treating their heroin addiction was relatively straightforward using methadone. The drugs I desperately struggled with, however, were the highly addictive diazepam and pregabalin, due to the very strict rules that I had to abide by when dealing with them.

Everyone had to be detoxed off them in prison, unless they could prove they were under specialist care and that they had been prescribed by a consultant within six months prior to being detained in custody.

Pregabalin is used to treat epilepsy, general anxiety disorder and neuropathic pain. Unfortunately, it has proved to be highly addictive and countless prisoners have told me that the withdrawal symptoms experienced, if they suddenly stop taking it, can be much worse than withdrawing from heroin.

Although some have it prescribed by their GPs outside, a great many also buy it on the streets, or off the internet, and take it in very high doses.

It has become highly tradable in prisons, so many will buy it from other prisoners, but if their supplier suddenly gets released or transferred to another prison, or gets moved to Separation and Care, then their supply is cut short. They would then suffer terrible withdrawals, and beg me for help.

Suzanne had been buying it on the wing, until her supplier had been released, and she was suffering from serious withdrawal symptoms, particularly overwhelming and crip pling anxiety.

'Please, Doctor Brown, please!' she begged, sounding desperate. 'I know I shouldn't have got myself into this mess, but I need you to help me out.'

I shook my head in despair. I hated seeing someone suffer but I couldn't break the rules. From the state she was in, it was obvious she wasn't faking it. She was shaking, sweating, crying.

I also knew her background, and that her anxiety stemmed from her fear of leaving prison; she was going to be homeless, and was frightened that she would be attacked or raped on the streets, as she had been in the past.

I had heard similar stories from so many women that I had no doubt it was true.

She was deeply insecure and emotionally fragile, and I appreciated her honesty in telling me that she had been buying it illicitly, so I made a deal with her. I agreed to prescribe it on the understanding that she would be detoxed off it, and that I would not be able to ever repeat this if she fell back into illicit use.

She agreed and thanked me profusely.

'But please don't conceal them and sell them,' I said. I could give her one chance and one chance only.

She nodded in agreement.

'Look after yourself, Suzanne,' I sighed.

'God bless you, Doc,' she replied.

*

I lifted the blind covering the small square window in the door, and peered through. There were at least a dozen women crowded outside my room in House Block One, shouting for my attention, but no nurse or officer.

Normally the nurse would be there to control the clinic, and to make sure that only patients on the list were seen at their appointed time.

'Doctor Brown!' one of the ladies shouted when she saw my face at the window. Then they all joined in. 'Doc, doc, I need you to see me today!'

I took a deep breath and opened my door.

'Have you all got an appointment?' I asked, almost certain that most of them hadn't. 'I'm really sorry, but if your name isn't on the list, I can't see you today.'

They weren't the sort to take no for an answer, hustling me until they got what they wanted. I swore under my breath.

Becky, the prison officer, spotted I was struggling. 'Break it up, girls,' she shouted, coming over to my rescue.

Becky was tough and very good at her job. Even though she was only 22, she had a 'don't mess with me' glare, and could easily have been mistaken for a bouncer on a nightclub door. She had short brown hair with a shaved undercut and several piercings – a bolt through her eyebrow and another through her tongue. Her facial features were elfin. She had beautiful big Bambi eyes and a tiny pixie nose.

She moved in front of my door, her arms crossed, her legs wide. 'If you haven't got an appointment, move on,' she barked.

'Thanks, Becky,' I said, before slipping inside the safety of my room. I leaned back against the door and sighed heavily. My shift hadn't even started and I was already feeling exhausted.

I logged onto the computer, but the drama continued to unfold outside my door.

'I'm not fucking moving until I see Doctor Brown,' a woman screeched. '*Doctor Brown!*'

'If you don't move away I'm going to dock your earned privileges.'

'Don't fucking speak to me like that, you dyke!'

'Right, that's it . . .'

All I could hear next was muffled cries, boots squeaking on the lino floor, and 'Get the fuck off me!'

The blinds rattled against the door as someone suddenly knocked on it.

I sighed. 'Who is it?'

'It's Rhianna. Rhianna James, Miss.'

I glanced down my list of names and saw that she was on it.

'Okay, come on in,' I said.

'There's a riot out there, Miss.' Rhianna closed the door warily.

She was a big woman, her arms were meaty and looked like they could throw a punch. She limped her way towards me, her lifeless straggly hair falling in front of her eyes.

She slowly lowered herself into the chair, keeping her right leg straight.

She had come to discuss her methadone, but there was clearly something wrong with her leg.

'How are you doing, Rhianna?' I asked, tentatively.

'Not good, Doc. 30mls of methadone is not holding me at all.'

I could see from her notes that she had arrived at Bronzefield three days ago, and that she was in and out of prison like a yo-yo. She told me that prior to custody she had been on a 70ml script, and so obviously her dose needed to be increased.

However, her main concern was a painful infected ulcer on her right lower leg, which emitted a very offensive odour that she was embarrassed about.

She fanned her hand trying to disperse the smell, and her cheeks turned scarlet. I asked her to pull up her trouser leg.

She was so embarrassed she could barely look at me. Slowly, Rhianna rolled up her grey tracksuit bottom, to reveal four sanitary towels stuck to her leg. The stench was beginning to engulf the airless room.

'It's all I could think of to dress it with,' she said, 'because I'm homeless and don't have a GP. I used them to absorb the pus, to try and stop it smelling so bad.'

A smell of rotting meat filled the room, forcing me to turn my head, catching myself from retching.

'I'm sorry.'

'No it's fine, Rhianna.' The nurse had arrived by then, and handed me some surgical gloves, and then managed to find some saline sachets and gauze. I started to gently peel off the sanitary towels, slowly, one by one. I held my breath as I did so. Lying underneath them was an extensive, deep infected ulcer just above the ankle, extending all the way up her lower leg.

The raw flesh was oozing pus and watery yellow fluids. The smell was revolting.

'Oh Rhianna, why haven't you tried to get help?' I asked.

Tears brimmed in her eyes. 'I was too embarrassed because of the smell.'

Her shame had stopped her seeking help.

The circulation in her leg had been compromised as a result of injecting in her groin, and so insufficient oxygen was getting to the skin, causing it to break down and allow the ulcer to form. She was already aware that she would have to stop injecting, as there was a risk in the longer term that she could end up losing her leg if she continued.

Rhianna wasn't alone in thinking she would be judged for the way she looked, the way she smelt, the fact she was homeless and took drugs. A lot of the women had told me that they felt ashamed of what they had become, and as a result didn't want to draw attention to themselves. They would rather suffer in silence, and some would risk death rather than ask for help.

I felt so desperately sorry for her, and for all the other homeless people out there.

I smiled. 'Don't worry, we will get you sorted. How long have you been using for?'

Rhianna looked to the ceiling as she searched for the answer.

'About fifteen years now, I reckon.'

We agreed a plan to get her stable on methadone, and I arranged for her to go straight over to Healthcare to get the ulcer cleaned and dressed in the wound clinic.

'Thank you so much,' she said, limping back out.

The thought of Rhianna sleeping rough in some doorway somewhere with that huge festering ulcer stayed with me well after she had left.

Unfortunately, so did the smell.

The thought of being stuck with it for the next couple of hours was dreadful, so I kicked off my shoes, clambered onto the chair and reached for the fan that was collecting dust on the top shelf.

I turned it on to full blast, in a desperate attempt to get the air circulating before the next patient arrived.

I picked up my mug to take a swig of coffee but one whiff of the combination of aromas was enough to turn my stomach. I placed it back down immediately, just as someone began banging on my door.

Chapter Twenty-Five

A lot of people in prison think they don't deserve to be there, but there are some who do. Amber was one such young woman.

She had recently been given a job working in Reception, helping the new residents when they arrived from court. She was a bright, articulate, pretty young lady, who was serving a staggering seventeen years for a crime I would have never guessed she would have committed. She was so sweet, and looked so innocent, it was difficult to think she had been convicted of handling firearms and supplying class A drugs, after becoming tangled up with the mafia.

But what surprised me most was how accepting she was of the harsh reality of spending the better part of the next two decades behind bars. That she would be in her mid-forties when she saw the world again.

'I deserve to be here,' she said, calmly, without a hint of self-pity.

Her case had been splashed all over the newspapers because of the length of her sentence. That, and the fact that she was a primary-school teacher who hid a machine gun in her knicker drawer.

She didn't seem the slightest bit fazed if people knew what she had done. and seemed much more focused on what she could do for others while she was inside.

Amber was training to be a trauma counsellor, so she could help support the residents in Bronzefield who had suffered physical and emotional abuse.

She had popped into my room for a quick chat while I waited for the next patient to be escorted to my door. It was always good to see her, as she was unfailingly cheerful and positive, and never seemed to feel sorry for herself. It was lovely to be able to chat as friends, rather than to always be seeing people in a clinical role.

She had thick, dark, glossy hair past her shoulders, beautiful big brown eyes, and a wonderful smile.

'If anyone asks what I've done, I tell them to Google me. I don't mind if they know.' She shrugged, nonchalantly. 'Acceptance is key. If you want to survive prison you have to come to terms with what you've done and the time you'll be in here,' she stated, matter-of-factly.

I agreed. I found that those who could not accept their situation struggled a lot more. So many prisoners asked for medication to ease their anxiety, their stress, their insomnia, because they were struggling to cope with being in prison. Like Azar, in the Scrubs, they struggled to accept where they were and the situation they found themselves in.

Those who had an 'I did the crime, so I'll do the time' attitude appeared to cope a lot better.

I also admired the fact that Amber was honest about

knowing what she was getting into when she met her husband, who had been sentenced to eighteen years for his part in the crimes.

She had grown up in a wealthy family on the outskirts of London, and she'd had everything she could ever have wanted as a child. Her life of luxury had continued when she'd married a man who was part of the mafia.

Reflecting on the past ten years, she said, 'I lived the mob-wife lifestyle in terms of the houses we lived in, the cars we drove.'

I was very curious as to how someone like Amber could have become mixed up with a mob family.

She smiled, her big brown eyes sparkling with the memory of meeting her man, who she was clearly still in love with.

'I had just completed my PGCE teacher training, when I first met him. It was a blind date arranged by friends of friends I'd known from my course. It really was love at first sight.' She blushed.

I offered her a biscuit as I usually had some in my bag to share around.

'Thank you,' she said, biting into the chocolate-covered biscuit. 'We were texting non-stop after that first night. A year and a half later, we moved in together.'

'So did you know who your husband really was?' I asked.

'At that point I kind of knew what he did,' she said, dabbing the crumbs from the corner of her mouth. 'But I didn't realise who he was. But when I met his family I was able to join up the dots, and his friends set me straight.'

'And that didn't bother you?'

She shook her head. 'No.'

Assuming I might be shocked by such a statement, Amber went on to elaborate. 'I was very independent and I wasn't interested in his money. I fell in love with who he was when he was with me, not the mafia character he was portrayed to be.

'What can I say? I just fell in love.'

In a strange way, it was sort of heartwarming to hear. I asked if he was older than her.

'He's six years older,' she replied.

To some young girls, I supposed, a successful rich older man with a dangerous side could be attractive.

'But,' she argued, 'I wasn't some young naïve girl. I knew who I married.'

'So you think you should be in prison?'

Without hesitation, Amber said, 'One hundred per cent I should be. Even though I wasn't dealing or involved, I knew we had drugs in the house, I knew that we had guns in the house, I was aware of what was going on. I was complicit, and that's why I'm here.'

She looked young, but she came across as much older than her 28 years.

Because of her lengthy sentence, she was located on House Block Four, where other prisoners with long-term sentences were also living, such as those serving time for murder, sex crimes, arson, manslaughter and terrorism.

'Do you think you were given an unfairly long sentence though? Some murderers get less?' I asked.

'Firearms are very dangerous, and what with everything that's going on in the world now . . .' She paused for a moment to consider her answer. 'Yes, I think my sentence was fair, we should have been made an example of.'

It was an extraordinary thing to admit to. I wondered if that was why she was training to be a counsellor, as a way of trying to pay society back for her crimes. She talked more about the training she was undergoing, and her desire to help others, seeming to read my mind when she said, 'I'm not doing it to make myself feel better. I do it because I want to make a difference and I know I can help these women.'

I learned that Amber had also been working as a 'listener', which is similar to the wonderful work the Samaritans do. She was on standby twenty-four hours a day to lend an ear to anyone who was struggling. That might mean going to see a prisoner in their cell in the middle of the night. I could imagine that she would make an excellent listener, as she had such a calm, kind, pragmatic way about her.

'Thank God I haven't been a victim of domestic violence, like so many of the poor women in here,' she said. 'But I've seen with my own eyes how destructive it can be. I have a close friend who is trapped in a violent relationship. She's always making excuses for him. It's as if she has been brainwashed. I used to tell her to leave him, that she needed to put herself and her children first. What I should have done is just be there on the other end of the phone for her if she needed to talk. But I feel I let her down, and was not always as sympathetic as I could have been. I'm putting that right now, though, with the work I'm doing here. Being a listener, training to be a trauma counsellor, it's an opportunity for me to give something back.'

Just as Amber was one hundred per cent certain she deserved to be in prison, I was one hundred per cent certain she was being sincere about her desire to help others.

I also admired her because she wasn't complaining about her sentence, or about losing her lavish lifestyle.

On the contrary, she told me that it had made her realise that most of the things she had owned, she hadn't needed.

'It was a shock to the system, I'm not going to lie. But you suddenly realise how little you need to get by.'

She shrugged. 'I adapted very quickly. I didn't even cry. I still haven't cried once, since I've been in here. It's just not me. Crying won't get me anywhere. I have to move on, I have to manage.'

'What about your husband, will you stay together?'

Amber cracked a smile. 'It's funny, everyone in here asks me that same question. I married him knowing what he was, so my feelings for him aren't going to change now we're in prison. I'm very loyal, I take marriage very seriously.

'I'm also in jail,' she added. 'So I'm in the same situation as him.

'I can visit him at his prison every six months. We're allowed inter-prison phone calls – I can speak to him every month. And we can write letters, of course.

'We're good, everything is good between us,' she smiled.

It wasn't a conventional relationship. But then, what did that matter if they loved each other?

Suddenly, Amber rose to her feet. She'd done all the talking she'd needed to do, and I could see she felt better for having someone to chat with. So did I.

I realised I was quite privileged to have her open up to me, and I wondered if locking things up inside was her way of staying in control of her life.

She gave me one of her sweet smiles. 'Do you mind if I have one more biscuit?' she asked.

'No, not at all!'

I handed her the whole pack to share with the others.

'You've got a good heart, Doctor Brown,' she said, and then disappeared out of the door.

Chapter Twenty-Six

I found most of the women I was meeting in my regular Substance Misuse Clinic fascinating. Trudy was no exception.

For years, Trudy had managed to hold down a full-time job as a housekeeper, alongside maintaining a serious heroin addiction. She'd looked after the luxurious homes of an immensely wealthy Middle Eastern family, and for decades she stayed out of trouble, working long hours and keeping up the pretence that all was okay when really she was crumbling inside.

It was her first time in prison, and as she sat in the chair in my little room, I could see the relief on her face. Her tired, frail body almost melted into the seat with liberation, but her eyes were flat and emotionless, as if she had used up all her tears long, long ago.

She was in her mid-forties, but looked older. Her skin was blotchy and flaky around her nose. Her hair was dark and straggly and going grey. Her voice was husky from cigarettes, and she coughed harshly.

'I can relax now,' she said, smiling wearily.

It was still a strange thing to hear – that being in prison

was better than being free, but it was something I had heard before so many times it no longer surprised me. I suppose being addicted to drugs had been a life sentence in itself for her.

And then she said something that left an impression on me. There was no window in my room, but Trudy gazed ahead, wistfully, as if she was imagining the most beautiful of views.

'I just want to live abroad, on a boat. I don't want anything else.'

Her words reminded me of the seascape that used to hang in my surgery, with a couple relaxing in the sunshine, looking out across a beautiful deep blue sea. When I felt like the world had got on top of me, I used to stare at that picture and wish I could just step into the frame, like Mary Poppins did in the film.

'Don't we all?' I smiled back.

She told me that she used drugs primarily to obliterate the memories of her abuse.

'At first my partner would make sure he hit me where no one would see. He would smack me in the stomach. The ribs. I was working with three broken ribs at one point.'

'He would hit me across my back with anything he could get his hands on, sometimes even the frying pan, or the saucepan.

'But the longer I was with him the less he cared about what people thought, so he started punching me in the face.'

'Oh goodness,' I sighed.

'I got good at using make-up. Concealer around my eyes, lots of foundation.

'It didn't really cover the black eyes, but nobody said anything to me. You wouldn't, would you? And a lot of the time my employers weren't living in the houses; they were abroad while I looked after them.'

She paused, suddenly considering what she'd just admitted. She frowned, crossing her arms defensively. 'I never stole from them if that's what you're thinking. Never once. I wouldn't do that. I was working all those hours so I could pay for myself.'

I quickly intervened. 'That's not what I'm thinking, Trudy. And I want you to know, I'm not here to judge you.'

She softened. 'I know, Doc. You seem like a good sort. I just didn't want you to think badly of me.'

'Well, I don't.' I smiled. It was funny how many of the women in Bronzefield seemed much more concerned about how I viewed them than the men in the Scrubs had been. I wondered if that sometimes had something to do with them needing me more, emotionally.

'So how did you end up with such a horrible partner? Did you try to leave him?'

'So many times, so many I lost count!' She spat the words out of her mouth.

'But he threatened to kill me if I left, and I was scared. By the end I'd given up, it was easier not to fight him any more. There was also a part of me that thought I couldn't do any better. He'd ground my confidence down so much, over the years. When I looked in the mirror I hated myself . . .' Trudy's voice started to wobble. Her face tensed.

'I hated my hair, my face, my body. I looked old and tired and covered in bruises, and who would want to be with someone who looked like that?'

She looked directly at me with sad, sad eyes. 'Who would want me?'

It was heartrending.

She wouldn't be the first woman afraid to be alone. Glancing back to Trudy's notes, it looked as if she had grown up around abuse. But I didn't need to ask. Trudy was a clever woman, and had already processed her reasons for putting up with the beatings.

'I suppose I knew no better. My dad was an alcoholic. He used to do a right number on my mum, couldn't even recognise her after he was done with her. He tried drowning her, he beat her with a poker, it was horrendous. And when he wasn't beating her, he would rape her in front of me and my sisters. He tried to kill my mum four times before she left him.'

What can you say to something like that? It was so far removed from the happy family life I'd grown up with. It's horrible to think that while you're getting hugs from your mum and your dad, someone somewhere else is watching their mum being beaten within a breath of her life. But that is life. And thanks to working in prisons, I finally had my eyes opened to what really goes on out there.

'It didn't stop there,' Trudy explained. 'Mum remarried not long after. She thought she had a good man in Carl, but he turned out to be just as bad as my dad. I was four when he first started touching me.'

'Oh, Trudy.' I shook my head in despair.

'Yeah, it was pretty bad, but I didn't know any better, you know? And my mum thought everything was okay because when I went up to bed I'd say, "Goodnight dad", as if he was my real father. As if I was happy.

'It was my fault for not speaking up.'

I quickly cut in. 'It wasn't your fault. You were only a child.'

Trudy pulled her sleeves over her hands, nervously.

'I should have told her, but I really thought it was normal. I thought rape, and violence, was just how families were.

'It moved from touching to full sex and I begged him to stop because he was hurting me. That's when he turned violent. He would hit me and threaten me. He said for every time I tried to stop him, he would beat my mum.'

Her voice cracked. 'What could I do?

'So I just let him.'

She looked down at her hands, tugged her sleeves, fighting the fabric that wouldn't stretch any further.

And then, with venom in her eyes, she said, 'When he was bored of me, he started bringing his friends around.'

Horrified, I clutched my hand over my mouth.

'He kept me off school so his friends could come over when my mum was out. She was working three jobs to keep us all.

'They took it in turns.' She paused. Then, her voice so low, so dead, she said, 'They all had a go, Doc.' She snorted. 'Well, what doesn't kill you makes you stronger.'

She shrugged and stared at the ground.

'Did you ever have counselling?' I asked.

'Nah.'

'Did you ever tell anyone what happened to you?'

'Yeah,' she replied, with disdain. 'I told my ex, the fella who beat me up for all those years. I was high one night, and feeling vulnerable, and finally opened up to him. I thought he would be there for me.'

'But he wasn't?'

'Was he hell! He just used it against me. Every time I ran away after he beat me up, he threatened that if I didn't come back, he would tell my sister that her dad was a paedophile. I didn't want to hurt my sister, because Carl had never touched her. I was terrified she wouldn't want to know me any more, and she was pretty much all the family I had left.

'And do you know the worst bit of it all is, Doc?' Trudy said.

'It wasn't the beatings, it wasn't the abuse. It was the fact that later in life, my mum got back together with my real dad. I was so angry we had gone through all of that pain and abuse for nothing.

'Nothing!' She spat out the words

We both sat in silence for a moment. I could see there was still a lot of hurt and anger buried within Trudy.

'Are you still with your partner now?' I asked.

'No, I finally left him. I also found the courage to tell my mum what happened to me.'

'What did she say?'

'She just feels really guilty. Says she didn't know, but I

think she didn't want to see it. I don't hate her for it, though. I understand she was abused too.'

She fell silent for a moment, looking off to one side, thinking. Then, the last thing I would have ever have imagined: a huge smile spread across her face.

'The most wonderful thing is that I finally found love. Real love. I have hope of a future. I'm so pleased to be in prison. To have a chance to get clean. I know you won't believe me, Doc, but I'm happy to be in here. I can stop pretending. It's over.'

She shook her head and said it again. 'It's over.'

That same look of relief Trudy had when she first sat down, washed back over her. She stopped tugging at her sleeves, she stopped scowling – her body relaxing.

'This is my chance to get myself off the drugs. To get *me* back.

'Will you help me Doc?'

It was music to my ears. 'Of course I will. How long do we have?'

'Eighteen months. I was using so much I'd got myself into debt, and I ended up dealing because I couldn't face the alternative.'

I knew what she was going say.

'I take my hat off to the girls who sell their bodies, but I couldn't do it. Not after everything I'd been through. I just couldn't.'

I nodded understandingly. I knew the story only too well.

'Yeah, hats off to them, but I couldn't.'

I began tapping away on my keyboard. 'So what are we going to do with your methadone?'

Before coming into prison, Trudy had been on a 70ml script, and was using heroin on top of that. Clearly, she had a big habit. We agreed a slow detox plan, as she had plenty of time. I also reassured her that if she was struggling at any point we could slow things down even further.

Trudy nodded politely. 'I was hoping you would say that. I don't want to do it fast. I have over a year to get off it.'

As she got up to leave, she suddenly remembered something.

'I almost forgot!' Trudy exclaimed. 'I'm seeing a psychiatrist and she has diagnosed me with post traumatic stress. I'm going to a trauma group every Friday. It's nice because there are other ladies in there who have been through similar stuff to me.'

'I am so happy for you, Trudy,' I smiled.

'A lot of people used to come to me with their problems, because I'm an easy-going person. I talk to anyone. I listen. Now, finally, it's me that's getting some help,' she said,

Suddenly, she lurched forward and wrapped her arms around me. In that brief moment that we hugged I could feel the happiness pour out of her. It was sad that Trudy saw prison as her only sanctuary, but at the same time I could see determination in her eyes – something I'm sure she wouldn't have had if she hadn't been sentenced to Bronzefield.

'You're such a lovely person,' I said. 'It's incredible how you functioned through all that horrific abuse, and the thought of you ending up on a lovely little boat somewhere fills me with joy.'

Trudy burst into laughter. 'I can see myself diving for shellfish. A little dog sitting on the end of the boat.' Flashing me a smile, she added, 'And my hunky man on the beach, fixing things.'

She carried that smile with her out of my door, and I was left feeling hopeful, too. I had over a year to help Trudy wean herself off methadone and, combined with the counselling, there was every chance she could leave Bronzefield with no drugs in her system, and no desire to go back on them when she returned to society. It was my goal to make her dream become a reality.

It was at that moment, that very second, that I realised I had reached my happy place. I had never had so much job satisfaction in all of my life. My journey to get there had been colourful, but I couldn't have been more fulfilled.

I felt and hoped that I was making a difference to these women's lives, which gave me joy and a sense of purpose. And as long as I was needed, and I was making a difference, I would carry on working as doctor, as a counsellor and also, hopefully, as a friend to these women.

There was a knock on my door. A nurse popped her head in. The screaming, the shouting, the swearing from the prisoners outside, came in with her.

'I've got your next patient here, Doc,' she said.

I smiled. 'Show her in.'

Acknowledgements

As I approach my 65th birthday, I am often asked by friends when I plan to stop work. The answer is always the same: when I stop enjoying it. The trouble is I don't think I ever will!

But, finally, when I do reach the end of my working road, and reflect on a lifetime of meeting and caring for hundreds of the most wonderful, fascinating people, from every possible walk of life, I will be at peace in the knowledge that the journey had been a truly magnificent one.

Thanks to Trudy, and to so very many of the wonderful women I have been lucky enough to meet and come to know in Bronzefield in the past few years. Trudy came to say goodbye to me before transferring to an open prison, after having successfully detoxed, and had transformed into a beautiful, confident woman. We had arrived at the end of our journey and embraced each other. She whispered, 'You've been wonderful, I could never have done this without you.' I feel that, just occasionally, I may have made some lives a little better. I am so grateful to everyone for that gift.

I would also like to thank my wonderful husband David

for his never-ending love, support and belief in me. My beloved sons Rob and Charlie for the joy, love and purpose they bring to my life, and to my dearest sister Laurie for the lifelong memories and love we share.

Many thanks to Susan Smith and Rachel Kenny for their support and belief in this project. I would also like to thank Ruth Kelly and Guy Adams for their help in telling my story, Kate Fox and Ben McConnell, my editors, for their constant encouragement and guidance.

I have met wonderful people who have enriched my working life. Of special note are Paula and Siobhan who made working at Huntercombe such fun. Jas and Denise for sharing the good and the bad times at The Scrubs. Harriet and Dayna from Bronzefield who both kindly took pity on me and helped type out passages of the book when my fingers were tiring.

Lastly, to my wonderful friend Vanessa who has listened patiently to my stories over the past twenty-two years and encouraged me to write this book.

And thank you for reading this.